Kids Sleep Meditation

A Complete Collection of Stories to Help Children Reduce Stress and Anxiety, Learn Mindfulness Meditation and Go to Sleep Feeling Calm, Happy and Confident

LILLY ANDERSEN

Tables of Contents

Introduction

This book focuses on helping your children feel great about themselves, relax, and prepare for a good night's sleep. There are numerous tips in each meditation to help your children comfort themselves before starting to meditate and some tactics at the end of every script for them and you as their guardian. Most of the time, taking a few minutes at the end of meditation to speak about thoughts, emotions, or feelings that came up can be vital in helping your kids relax further before going to bed. Try to put aside at least five minutes after each meditation process to talk with your children about how they are feeling. You could ask them if anything came up that they want to tell you.

Children as young as three years have been known to benefit substantially from meditation sessions practiced regularly. Children who experience these meditation exercises plan tasks better and have a better memory. Moreover, they have the perfect ability to organize information as opposed to their peers. Additionally, meditation scripts have also been found to be vital in children dealing with fears they start to develop in their younger years. For instance, things like being afraid of monsters or darkness, or emotional worries, such as fear of not being perfect or fear of being left alone can all be dealt with by practicing meditation regularly.

To enjoy the most from this meditation exercise, advise your children to find a place in the house or wherever they are listening to these meditations where they can relax and settle down. It does not need to be the same place every time, but having a regular meditation routine helps their body start relaxing faster the more they repeat their meditation patterns. Tips on how to settle in before the meditation sessions are offered at the start of each chapter to help remind you and your child to start the relaxation process, but try to think of some now before you get started, so you feel prepared and ready for the first meditation.

A significant number of kids suffer from some form of sleep inadequacy. As earlier presented, depriving yourself of sleep will lead to poor concentration and irritability among others. The dangers of inadequate sleep can include depressed enjoyment of life and dangerous driving. Sleep insomnia occurs in two main forms which include one where you have difficulties falling asleep and where you have challenges resuming sleep after waking up. Fortunately, as seen hypnosis, guided imagery and guided meditation can help combat all forms of insomnia.

Remember that if you wake up in the night with thoughts going through your mind you are having a night of disrupted sleep. The mind is still active and cannot let the whole body rest when there is a pending business. Meditation is thus meant to help ease off these activities needs in your mind to help achieve threshold relaxation levels. One of the best approaches to trigger sleep meditation is to count the breaths you take. Begin the preparation to sleep meditation any scanning through your body and searching for areas of relaxation and tension. Now start counting breaths that are each inhalation and exhalation up to ten. The mind may wander but invite it back to the counting of breaths exercise. The goal is to shift away from the worrisome thinking and grant the mind a different object to focus on while the mind wanders off.

The Chaos in Magic

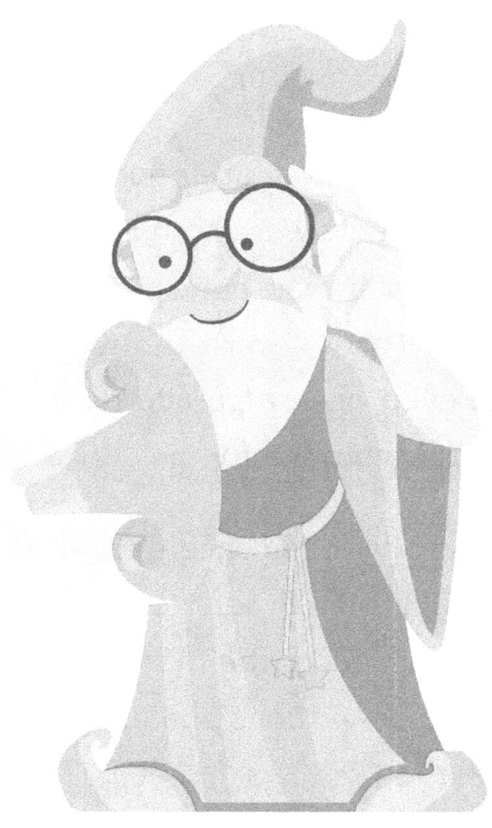

Hemlock always seemed to have the deck stacked in his favor. He was a handsome young wizard living in Spindle, one of the few mortal villages in Whimsy. Born to nobility, he was given an exceptional private education. His mother and father both had magical abilities, something that they'd passed down to their only son. Such powers were not the norm in his area.

The human villages were the most reminiscent of the Earth realm, during the era of the Victorian queen. The occupants knew of the mystical creatures beyond their borders, but as mostly defenseless humans, they did their best to segregate themselves from the rest of their world. For this reason, those with magic were fascinating to the population of Spindle. Those with gifts were given instant celebrity status.

Hemlock began receiving this extra attention from the moment he was born. His parents were both revered and famous. The birth of their son was anticipated by the villagers, well in advance. Parties were thrown for his arrival. There may have even been a parade right down the most central road of this community.

Hemlock's mother was the only one concerned with how this intense intrigue might affect her son. She was terrified of him becoming spoiled by the mass interest in him. She wanted her son to be virtuous and humble, and for the most part, he was. At first.

In the throes of his early childhood, he was kept oblivious to his own popularity. His mother homeschooled the young wizard, his public outings to nonexistent. She was so intent on keeping his head level, that she accidentally isolated her son. His mother also somewhat selfishly, wanted to keep her beautiful son beside her always. She wanted to shield him from the influences of fame. This was a completely unsustainable plan, but she treasured her child and would do anything to keep him safe.

 Hemlock was a lonely boy, using his free time to further develop his magical abilities. His mother emphasized the necessity of keeping his identity secret. He longed for a friend, looking for someone else that could empathize with his plight.

Meanwhile, outside of the oppressive walls of his family's small mansion, the whole village was constantly lit up with rumors about the identity of the magical son. A mass curiosity that did not fade much with time.

Eventually, the need for companionship became so great that he began to sneak out of his gated family home when his parents were away. The village of Spindle knew of Hemlock's existence, but they had never seen his face. Being kept from the public eye allowed him to create a new persona for himself, to be used during these adventures. He called himself Herb and dressed as a member of the working class, as to not arouse suspicion.

He was jealous of the mortals and their sense of community. Every young villager roamed around with friends, something that Hemlock had never experienced. He watched from the shadows as they laughed and played among themselves. The envy gave way to a longing that created a deep ache within his soul. Their smiles were so free and natural.

It was during one of these outings that our hero was stumbled upon by a young lady from the village. She looked to be around the same age as Hemlock, which at the time was seventeen. By then, he had been wandering through public as Herb for years and years. He was well-practiced in avoiding attention by blending into the background of bustling mortal life. So, what could have changed about this day, you ask?

As Hemlock sat on a bench at the edge of a quiet garden park watching the people pass, he was spotted by a friendly dog that had only just slipped his owner. The canine approached the young wizard, looking for attention. His owner was close behind him, a mortal named Charlotte.

She ran as fast as she could in an effort to keep her dog off of the stranger, but alas, her pet was taken with the secret wizard and had jumped on his lap. Hemlock loved dogs and had always wanted a pet for himself, but his father had always fought him on such issues, being less allergic and more just not a fan of pet hair. The young wizard stroked the animal's head as it gazed at him in adoration.

Upon reaching the two of them, Charlotte immediately apologized and began to explain that her dog had a tendency to slip his leash and run. She stopped midsentence, though, as she was taken by the presence of the handsome young stranger. Hemlock was a tall young man, with a mess of brown curls atop his moon-shaped face. He had this look of innocence, courtesy of his round cheeks. He shared an icy pale eye color with his mother.

Charlotte introduced herself to Hemlock, who, of course, told her that his name was Herb. He could not help but feel very comfortable speaking to the young lady, as she had a very warm and inviting nature. He thought that she and her dog fit rather well together.

As the two sat together and talked, Hemlock did his best to keep the lying to a minimum. Anytime Charlotte would ask him questions about his past or family, and he would do his best to redirect the conversation. The pair bonded on that park bench for hours. He agreed to meet her there the next day so that they might further enjoy one another's company. Hemlock had never so candidly spoken to a stranger, and the whole experience left the wizard feeling lighter than air. In fact, he awoke from a dream that night to find himself floating above his bed. He only wished that he could be completely honest with her about his life.

Hemlock (or "Herb") continued to meet Charlotte in that park every opportunity that he got. Sometimes, he would even use his magic to shoot a suggestion to the young lady that she should really go and walk her dog. To spite Charlotte knowing about the wizard's true nature, the two became best friends. To Hemlock, she was his only and most important friend.

Charlotte was a short and spunky young woman with bright and lovely features. Long black hair fell around her slender face in waves. She had a nose that pointed up at the end, like what those in the Earth Realm might call a ski slope. Her large gray eyes had captivated Hemlock from the moment he made her acquaintance. He was hopelessly smitten with his first and only friend but knew that he would never ever risk their bond for romance. Hemlock had mostly resigned to never knowing a mutual love. His favorite this about Charlotte was not her huge eyes or dainty and comical face, but the fact that she didn't hold back her feelings at all. Even when her opinions were in stark contrast to his own, she proudly spoke her piece. She was both calm and respectful. When the friends disagreed on a topic, neither would take the other's differing views personally. She was unlike anyone else in his life in that way. He had no idea yet, but he would come to value this even more in the coming months.

As time wore on, Charlotte introduced Hemlock to her family. He would often come and visit with them, sometimes even in her absence. Sneaking out of his own house was becoming more and more difficult, so he told his parents that he must commune with nature for hours every day, to keep his abilities sharp. In her family, he found an acceptance that he had never known anywhere else. He was loved and listened to and treated like any other relative. Their small brick house became his haven away from the expectations of his own family. His own parents loved him to death, too, but they were aloof and unaffectionate by nature. Charlotte's family was open and warm.

Hemlock had almost slipped up by using magic in front of Charlotte on several occasions, especially because the young lady was clumsy and accident-prone. He could not just watch her fall without intervening, thankfully Charlotte was very trusting and always found a way to explain any particular movement of objects or her own falling body, away. She slowly became very impressed by both her luck and the power of regular wind.

It is so easy to get carried away by your own desires. It is easy to become intoxicated by the universe, seemingly granting your most secret wishes. Hemlock being accepted by Charlotte's family, was a catalyst for him. He wanted them to know everything about him. He didn't want to hide his nature from her anymore either. He wanted the whole village to see him for the talented young wizard that he was. His magic was a large part of him, and he felt so much guilt from not being able to share it with the people that he had come to love. The longing to be honest with everyone was slowly eating away at his thoughts. He began formulating a plan.

On an unusually chilly August day, Hemlock transmitted a subconscious thought to Charlotte. She should go and walk her dog today after all this seemed to be the maiden breath of autumn (her favorite season). Hemlock's parents happened to be in town on this day, for what the village referred to as The Augustine Fair.

It was just one of many celebrations held in the large park at the center of the village; the same park where their son had first met his only friend. Hemlock picked this day for one important reason. It was the day of his birth, eighteen years ago. He was now an adult, and he would use this as a means by which to finally meet his peers. His mother would never have approved of his idea, but he refused to stay hidden forever. Hemlock could not be anonymous for the rest of his life, and he had no idea how much longer his parents would insist on keeping his face a secret from their community.

His parents both donated to and participated in the event. Proceeds were gifted to the less fortunate. It was a large festival with games, singing, talent acts, rides, and food. Hemlock's parents would perform feats of magic before their adoring fans, such as levitating audience members and performing acts of disappearance. The crowd favorite was a stunt that included his mother raising a perfect orb of fire above her head. Those who had watched their performance were always left speechless.

When Hemlock arrived at the large park, Charlotte was already there with her dog. He rushed to meet her, embracing her. This took her by surprise, as they had never hugged before. She blushed as the young wizard held her for a moment that passed too quickly. Hemlock pulled back and thanked her for meeting him here. She was understandably confused because the idea of walking her dog seemed to like her own. She was so pleased to see her closest friend, though, that she quickly brushed off the sentiment.

She was shocked by his dapper change in attire; he looked mysterious and otherworldly. He was wearing dark high collared shirt, vest, and jet-black trousers. His coat was also a crisp looking contrast to what he normally wore. His bowtie was the only pop of color within the outfit, and even that was a deep navy blue. He also wore a top hat, which lent even more to the sophistication in his appearance that day. These clothes seemed to compliment his personality much more than his usual loose brown vest and coat. He looked like an outwardly different person, but once Charlotte caught sight of his familiar facial expressions, she knew that he was still just regular Herb.

"I am so glad that you're here! I had completely forgotten that Augustine was today. We can walk around and make a real day of it. I just love the fair." Charlotte said.

"That sounds like the perfect birthday present! I have one thing that I must do first, though. I'd like you to promise me that you won't be furious at me for keeping a secret from you. It doesn't change anything; you know me more than anyone else. I was forced by circumstance to make a very difficult choice and today is the day that I rebel against all this unnecessary mystery. I know that your first instinct will be to hate me for misleading you. I just want you to understand that you and your family have made all the difference in my life. You are the reason I want to be honest." Hemlock said, his hands shaking from fear.

"It's your birthday!? Happy birthday, Herb! Is that your secret? Why didn't you tell anyone? I could never hate you." Charlotte said, confused but with a giant grin on her face.

"Well, it is my birthday, but I can only wish that were my secret. Today I am going to show you who I really am." A single tear ran down the young wizard's face as his chest rose and fell rapidly. This was going to be the scariest moment of his life so far. Seeing his distress, Charlotte threw her arms around him again and whispered to him that everything was going to be alright. She told him that no matter what happened, she would always be here when he needed her. This brought a measure of comfort to the terrified young man, and he did his best to slow his frantic breathing back down. Hemlock turned around just in time to see his parents walk out onto a large wooden stage that had been assembled for the event, in the center of the park.

"Aren't they amazing? What I wouldn't give to have magic. They are the most graceful looking couple that has ever existed. Did you know that they supposedly have a son our age? No one has ever seen him; some people don't even believe that he exists." Charlotte said while staring wide-eyed at his parents as they levitated an audience member. "They're so perfect that they don't even seem real. They're too beautiful. The magic, the wealth; they have everything. I bet they hate doing events like this with us regular folks." As Charlotte was saying these words, Hemlock felt his heart fall to his stomach once again. He could have thrown up. "I...if you were to ask them, I bet they would tell you... this is probably the only fun engagement that they have this month." Hemlock said, choking on his words.

"Their idea of fun has to be much more sophisticated than ours!" Charlotte laughed.

"You would be surprised." Hemlock smiled weakly.

"What? How on Whimsy could you know?" Charlotte asked.

"Surprise!" Hemlock said with an unsteady voice as he turned and began marching toward the stage.

The first to see him was his mother. She accidentally released the mortal that she was levitating, and they fell two feet to the ground. Hemlock watched as his mother's eyes widened in shock and her mouth gaped open. He noticed that she had a look upon her face as though she were doing a very complex math equation in her head. Then, in an instant, her expression changed to one of resignation. A calm seemed to wash over her features, and she smiled at her son. His father made eye contact with his son, and it was the most unusual thing... a look of pride. He had always secretly wanted to show off his son to the village but refrained out of respect for his wife. His father was beaming as his son made his way onto the small stage. The young man was so nervous that it felt as if his heart was trying to beat its way out of his chest.

"Attention, everyone! It is my sincerest pleasure to introduce to you, our son Hemlock." His father roared happily to the audience. He wrapped an arm around the young wizard, and a hush fell over the audience. Then thunderous applause.

The whole village had been waiting to meet Hemlock from the moment he was born. His mother wrapped her arm around him from his opposite side. "Would you like to see what he can do?" His father asked the crowd, and they responded enthusiastically. He then whispered to his son, making sure that he had prepared a stunt for his grand takeover of the stage.

Hemlock held his arms out in front of his body at a downward angle. As he rose them to be level with his shoulders, a ball of water began to form above his head. His mother took the hint and joined in his performance with her crowd favorite fireball. The two of them must have had the same idea because, in tandem, they began to move these orbs closer together. A loud and satisfying crackling occurred as the two forced joined and then disappeared into nothing. The hordes of onlookers went mad for this demonstration, clapping for the pair with an addictive intensity. The family then joined hands and bowed.

Hemlock had never experienced a feeling like this before. So many people cheered him on, and that sort of approval was something that never crossed his mind. His had been a life of blending into the background, until now. This new feeling lit a fire in his soul and spoke to a part of him that he didn't know existed.

Following the performance, the young wizard pushed through the jumble of fans in the park, looking for

Charlotte. He found her right where he left her before the show. She looked positively shocked. So many emotions this young woman was trying to account for, all at once. She was furious that he had kept his identity a secret from her, but part of her understood that it wasn't a choice he wanted to make. Charlotte was also astounded by his magic and pretty sure that she was in love with him. She also felt a disconnect now, as though he and his family were miles above her. How could she even speak to him now? The thought of it made her knees feel weak. Hemlock? His name wasn't even really Herb! Goodness though, 'Hemlock' was a purely magical word.

She snapped out of her daze when the young wizard embraced her again. He was apologizing profusely and saying over and over again, that he was still the same man. His hug melted away all the angst that she had felt only a moment ago. It would take time, but Charlotte would forgive him. It helped that he explained the reason for his disguise was his own mother; he was trying to keep her from knowing about his sneaking out. Charlotte eventually came to sympathize with the story of his lonely childhood.   The pair slowly repaired their friendship, and he was finally able to be completely honest about her. The transmitting of subconscious thoughts was one of the few points of contention after a while. She eventually even gave in and forgave him for that too, because it happened to be extremely useful. Charlotte told him that he needed to make it known from now on when he sent her a thought. None of this is making her think things were her ideas when they were obviously not. She considered that to be an invasion of her privacy. Her family was also very forgiving of the young wizard, and eventually, he was able to bring his own parents to meet and visit with his second family.

The adoration from strangers in the village was a huge adjustment for Hemlock. They perused him, asking for magical favors or a demonstration of his power. He didn't mind any of this, because he was so grateful to finally be seen as himself and not Herb. He would not admit it to anyone, but he loved the attention. Hemlock had been ignored by the public for as long as he could remember, and now it was like he was a king or an Earth Realm Rockstar roaming among his fans. Slowly he began to crave their interest in him. Little by little his ego was growing. Just as he was getting used to being loved for who he was, his magic began to go haywire. It was just little glitches at first, but of course, it got worse. Sometimes he would go to light a match with his mind, and he would incinerate an object near him instead. Hemlock was content to write it off as growing pains and ignore the issue until something happened that he could not ignore.

One afternoon while practicing, the young wizard accidentally set himself on fire. Luckily, he had already developed the water trick and was able to put it out immediately, even if he was soaked now. What if that had been someone else, though, what would he have done? His mind blinked back to Charlotte, what if he had hurt her. He would never forgive himself. Hemlock was pretty sure that he was in love with his best friend, which is a thought that he absolutely did not mean to transfer to her. His eyes widened, and he felt his heart fall into his stomach.

The fire had been nothing compared to accidentally bearing his soul to Charlotte. How would he ever face her now? The thought had sent, he felt it. He knew that it had to have gone to her. She had to know now. What if he just pretended that nothing happened? What if he ignored it?

He ran to his mother and begged to know why his powers were rebelling against him. She told him that he might be too wrapped up in the attention that he is receiving from is gifts. She mentioned that the universe always seems to know when you are misusing magic, and it has some pretty cruel ways to get back at you. He could feel himself blushing at her words. He asked his mother if there was any way that he could potentially rewind time?

"No, but you can meditate and find meaning in your magic again. That way, nothing else will happen. You need to be in this for the right reasons. If you can't handle the attention that being a wizard brings you, without your ego growing, then you need must step away from the public eye. Or learn to humble yourself. Do you want to talk about what happened with your magic?"

"No, I really don't. Thank you so much for the advice, though. I will find a way to fix my intentions." Hemlock said, nervously.

"Meditation and breath control always worked for me!" Said his mother.

Hemlock tried meditating later that day. He felt as though the magic glitching and ruining his life had humbled him enough, but he wanted to make absolutely sure that he was not going to be walking around, just broadcasting his innermost feelings to people. Hemlock felt amazing after quieting his racing mind. He concentrated on his breathing so that he could get into the right frame of mind, and everything else came naturally.

He decided that he would take a few days away from the public eye for more than one reason. The young wizard was content to hide in his parent's lavish house. He was too ashamed to go outside. That is when he heard a knock at the front door, he scrambled from his bed and cracked the door to his room so he could see what was going on. His mother had answered it.

"Hey, Charlotte, so nice to see you. I will go and get him!"

Mary and Miranda

Miranda turned six years old when her father got her a hamster for her birthday. He told her that he found the 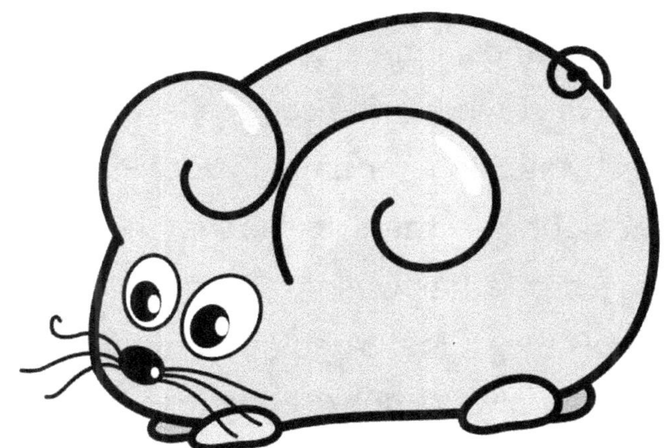 hamster on the street as if she were a stray cat. Miranda got many different presents that year, but this was her favorite one by far.

She wanted to spend all her time playing with this hamster she named Mary. They would run around together on the carpet, even though Miranda's father didn't like this at all. She still took Mary out of her cage and chased her around when he wasn't looking.

She tried to dress up Mary in her doll clothes, but the hamster didn't seem to like it. It didn't help that the clothes barely fit. Miranda's father came by a lot to check on them because he stopped trusting his daughter with her pet. He told her that hamsters are meant to stay in their cage, or else they might get sick.

But Miranda didn't see any fun at all in that. If Mary always stayed in the cage, she would only be able to pet her by sticking her hand inside. Plus, she figured it would get boring in there if she was never able to leave. Any time her father wasn't around, Miranda and Mary broke all of the rules, running around until they got tired. Miranda always got tired before the hamster did.

Mary never seemed happy to go back in the cage, which Miranda understood. If she was in a cage herself, she would not be happy, either. This was why she tried to take her out as much as possible.

Even when her father was home, Miranda played with her pet. She would read stories to her, mostly rhymes that she found in the library. Even Miranda got bored when she was read to sometimes, so she was surprised that Mary seemed interested in all of the stories. She stood at the edge of the cage and listened intently. T

the truth was, Miranda didn't even want to go to bed with Mary around. All of her other toys seemed boring now that she had Mary around. Her father made a big deal out of her birthday this year and got her all sorts of presents, but Mary was the only one that she cared about. She didn't even mind cleaning after her and feeding her, doing the things that her father said were teaching her responsibility. She would do anything for her pet.

Miranda had always said that she wanted a dog, but now she wouldn't want one, because she would be worried that it would hurt Mary. She even thought about Mary as she drifted off into sleep, thinking about all the fun things they would do together once she got up. Maybe tomorrow, they could play outside together. The possibilities were endless when the two of them spent time together because Miranda had a very good imagination.

Miranda had a lot of trouble falling asleep that night she got Mary, thinking about everything they would do the next day. She didn't even want to fall asleep. She wanted to get out of bed and think of the possibilities of what they could do, and then do them. Miranda was tossing and turning so much that she eventually got out of bed completely. She had to see what Mary was up to. Maybe she was having the same problem, and she couldn't get to bed either. Miranda walked over to the cage and gasped. Mary, the hamster, was completely gone. She didn't hear her scamper away or make any noise at all, so she must have been so distracted by her thoughts that she wasn't able to hear her. Quietly, she flipped on the switch in her room so her father wouldn't hear. She looked around everything to find her: under her bed, in her closet, in her toy box. Mary was nowhere to be found. She was nervous about leaving her room and waking her father up, but she didn't want to lose her hamster forever. This was urgent: Miranda had to find her right this instant.

Next, she checked the bathroom. Mary wasn't in the sink, cabinet, or the shower. She was frustrated that she couldn't check in her father's room without waking him because Mary was probably small enough to squeeze under the door. But she couldn't check there, so she went into the living room. She looked inside the entertainment center, under the table, and behind the couch. Her hamster wasn't here either. Then Miranda looked in the kitchen. She was starting to get nervous because there were only so many places that she could look. Even though she didn't know how she would get in there, she looked in the fridge last when she couldn't find Mary anywhere else. What if Mary went somewhere that she wouldn't even be able to reach? What if she went somewhere so dark and small that she would be impossible to find there? She tried to put these thoughts away. She checked under the dining room table. Nothing. Everywhere she checked, Miranda couldn't find her hamster.

Besides her father's room, there was only one more place where Mary could be: in the library. It was a small room in the back of the house with a few bookshelves. Her father was a big reader, so he liked to spend a lot of time in there. Sometimes he would even stay up late reading a book in there under a lamp, but thankfully that wasn't tonight, or Miranda would get caught being up late.

To Miranda's surprise, there was a lamp on, but it wasn't her father who was in there. In fact, she didn't see anyone at all. And it wasn't like her father to leave lights on.

The lamp wasn't where her father normally placed it,

either. It was where he picked it up from before he placed it on the end table next to his chair, but in this spot, it was on. Strangely, there was an open book placed next to it — and more strangely than that, she saw Mary on top of that book, looking down and staying still. Mary didn't even seem to notice that Miranda was there.

"Mary, what are you doing?" Miranda said. She could barely reach the shelf that Mary was on, but she looked up with her neck stretched far out to see her. "How did you get out of your cage without my help?"

Mary finally seemed to notice that her owner was there, as she stopped looking down at the page, and looked over to where Miranda was standing. Mary started to pace around on top of the book. She got a bookmark in her mouth and placed it on top of the page she was standing on.

"You're so funny, Mary. It looks like you're reading that book," she laughed. "I'm not a hamster, and even I can barely read right now. We are getting better at it in school, though. Oh, I wish I could take you to my school so we could spend all our time together! Then I wouldn't have to wait until I got home to play with you. Wouldn't that be fun?" Miranda asked.

Mary nuzzled her little hamster head to close the book she had been standing on top of. Miranda stretched up her hands as high as they could go so, she could grab the book Mary had appeared to be reading.

"Let's see what kinds of books you like," Miranda said, smiling. "*Storybook Classics*. I love this one! My daddy used to read it to me every night, but now he says I'm too old for it. He started reading me harder books that they give out in school, so I can read things a little harder than this one right now. Maybe one day, you'll be able to read chapter books too, Mary!"

Miranda put the storybook down on her father's end table, and she reached up again to take Mary into her hands.

"You really liked that last story I read you, didn't you?" Miranda said. "I'll be sure to read to you way more. When my daddy is around, we can't play outside your cage anyway, so that's a good time for me to read to you. Does that sound good to you?"

Miranda laughed again, knowing that her hamster

wouldn't be able to say anything. But for the second time that night, Miranda gasped, because her hamster started speaking.

"I would love to read more stories with you, Miranda," Mary said.

Miranda nearly dropped her hamster in surprised, but thankfully she got her balance back and put her down on her father's chair.

Miranda was still extremely surprised, and while she was a chatty girl, she had no idea what to say to Mary. She was used to talking to her a lot, but when she started speaking to her, it was completely different. She never thought Mary would actually say anything back.

"It's like in the movies!" Miranda exclaimed. But she realized she might wake up her father, so she tried to quiet down. "I have many questions for you. Is it like in the movies where all animals can talk to each other, or can you only understand only hamsters? Do you speak in a different language with hamsters, or do you speak English too? Am I the only person who can understand you and other people just don't listen? Or do you just not usually talk around people."

"I'm glad to have a friend like you with so many questions," Mary said. "I can give you answers, too. Well, I don't know how to talk to any other animals, actually. Even other hamsters. Animals don't really have a language they can speak to each other in the way that humans do. That's what makes humans so special. In fact, I'm the only animal I know who can talk. I wasn't always this way; it was just the environment I was in that taught me how to do it. You might say that I got smart from reading books and listening to people. If you read and listen as much as I do, you'll get smart, too."

"Wow, you sound like an adult talking," Miranda said. She was trying to keep her voice down now. "If you're so smart, why are you reading a book that even a kid like me is too young for?"

"You don't have to be a kid to enjoy kid's stories," Mary said. "I love reading stories meant for children. I like adult's stories too, but sometimes they don't have the same sense of wonder that comes with childhood. You'll understand when you get older. You know, C.S. Lewis said that when he was a kid, he used to read kid's stories in secret, but as an adult, he read them in the open."

"I don't know who C.S. Lewis is, but it sounds like you've read a lot of books," Mary said. "So, it's okay with you if I read books that are below your reading level?"

Mary laughed. Miranda was surprised at how much it sounded like a human laugh. "Of course, you can. I just told you, I still like children's stories a lot. They're a great place to learn lessons, and even adults need to learn lessons. I like to think of children's stories as stories that everyone can enjoy, not just as for kids. Everyone can enjoy children's stories and bond over them and learn the lesson together."

"You're saying that I could be as smart as you if I read as much?" Miranda asked.

"I think you're very smart already, but anyone can get smarter if they read more," Mary said. "I can help you get better at reading if you want, but you can't tell your father about how I can talk. A lot of adults get scared of things like that."

"Really? But you're not scary," Miranda said.

"You're a child, so it's different for you. Your father might not even let me live here anymore," Mary said.

Mary started to look sad, and Miranda could even tell with her little hamster face. Mary crawled back up to the top of the bookshelf so she could talk to her properly.

"There's something I want to talk to you about, though, Miranda," Mary said.

"What is that? You sound like something is the matter. Don't hold your feelings in, tell me what you are feeling," Miranda replied.

"It's about living here with you. I really love playing with you at your house, but your dad actually found me when I got lost from my old home," Mary said. She nibbled on some food that she had found on the carpet.

"Where did your owner live before?" Miranda asked.

It was a long story, but Mary told it to her new owner.

Mary used to be a class pet for a class of second graders. The teacher's name was Ms. Webb, but she wasn't the only owner. Every student took turns being responsible for Mary. Almost all of them were very sweet children, but there was one little boy named Charlie. Charlie was where all the problems started.

It was Charlie's job to take care of her that week and feed her. But he didn't do what he was supposed to do; he didn't follow the rules whatsoever. In fact, he tortured her more than he took care of her. He would poke and prod at her, causing her a lot of pain. He even refused to feed her because he thought it was funny.

Mary didn't want to talk badly about any of the students, even Charlie. She thought maybe he had problems going on at home that would cause him to act this way. Miranda couldn't understand why a kid would be so cruel, but after all the reading Mary had done, she knew how awful people could be.

The last straw was when Charlie started to come to Mary with a sharpened pencil. Mary didn't feel safe in that classroom anymore. It made her very sad, but she had to leave for her own safety. That was when Mary learned how to escape her cage without anyone else's help.

When Charlie came at her with the fork, she rushed into

the cage door and ran across the floor of the classroom. Charlie tried to chase her down, but he couldn't catch her in time. Mary ran through the hallway of the school, but she was so scared of the boy catching up with her that she just kept running.

Before she even knew it, Mary was outside in the playground. Kids were running across the field, and she was scared of getting stepped on, so she got out of there and went into the street.

Mary knew from books that roads were a dangerous place for a hamster, but it seemed like everywhere was dangerous for her. Miranda asked Mary what school she used to be in the classroom of, and Mary told her it was Ridgeland Park Elementary School.

"That's the elementary school I go to," Miranda said. "But I'm only in the first grade. I wish I could be in your class, but I'm too young. I'm really sorry about what happened with that mean little boy, Mary. I promise you most little boys aren't like that. I don't understand why he would be so mean to you."

"I know that most little boys are nice, Miranda. But I was

so scared, and I didn't know what to do, so I just ran away. I'm afraid that even if I go back, he'll still get his turn to take care of me, and he'll do the same thing. And that's what I actually want to ask you about, Miranda," Mary said. She stopped nibbling on the crumb and looked at her new owner with hamster eyes. "I want to go back home, but I need you to tell Ms. Webb about what happened with Charlie; that way, he gets punished, and I know that I can go back safely."

Miranda almost started crying. She didn't want to lose her new friend, right after she had just gotten her. She was filled with emotions, because she didn't want to take Mary away from the people who loved her, either. The students in Ms. Webb's class must have really missed their hamster, Mary.

"I'm sorry, Mary, but I just can't do it!" Miranda cried. She couldn't control her volume at this point, and it was surprising that she didn't wake her dad up. "I know you like being in the class with all those kids where you got really smart, but I don't want to give you away when we just became friends! I'm not even in the second grade, so I would never be able to see you. Maybe sometimes, but we wouldn't get to spend a lot of time together like we do now."

"You could still see me, Miranda," Mary said. She had expected Miranda to react this way, but she was still disappointed. It was a lost opportunity: she shouldn't have even let Mary catch her reading in the first place or let her hear her talk, but she figured if she had, she might as well try to get Miranda to bring her back home. "I understand that you want us to stay as friends, though. When I was a little hamster girl, I would have wanted the same thing. Don't worry about it. I can stay here with you, and you can be my new family, then. But for right now, you should probably go to bed. It's very late for a child your age."

Miranda was tearing up, but she was relieved when Mary said this. "Do you want to stay in here and read, or do you want me to take you back to your cage?"

Mary sighed sadly. "I'll go to bed. Don't worry about carrying me, though. I can get there by myself just like I got out. You definitely need to get to bed, though, Miranda. You have school in the morning, and it's nearly morning already."

Miranda did what she said and got under her covers. She has mixed feelings. She didn't want to lose her new friend already, but Mary seemed upset that she wouldn't go home. She didn't know what to do.

After that night, Mary didn't seem the same anymore. Miranda would take her out to play, but all she wanted to do was stay seated in the same spot and look down. She still talked to Miranda, but she didn't say much. Weeks went on like this, and Miranda felt like her friend wasn't the same as she was when she first got her as a pet.

She knew it was because she didn't take her to her old family, but the idea of losing Mary made her sad, too. It seemed like no matter what she did, either Mary would be upset, or she would be. Miranda wished there was a way she could make both of them happy without having to lose her.

But when the weather started to get warmer, Mary seemed to be in even worse shape than before. She barely ate any of the food she gave her, and she didn't talk to her as much as she used to. Miranda was at a loss. Did she have to let Mary go for her to be happy again?

She wasn't sure how she would help her, anyway. Her father didn't know that the hamster was originally someone else's, and she couldn't tell him that Mary could talk and that she told her about her last owner.

Miranda was lying in bed again, feeling really guilty about all of this. It was just like the first night after she got Mary, but this time she was tossing and turning out of worry, not because she was excited for the next day. Once again, Miranda got out of bed when she couldn't get herself to sleep — and once again, she looked in Mary's cage, assuming she would be gone and out in the library reading.

But Mary wasn't. She wasn't asleep, either, but she was still in her cage, looking sad.

"Why didn't you go read like you always do?" Miranda asked, stretching her arms out as she got out of her bed.

"I haven't been doing that in a really long time. I'm just not in the mood for it anymore," Mary said. She looked down like she did when she was reading, but she just looked sad. "It does make me really happy to be your pet, Miranda. You're the nicest, brightest little girl I've ever met. But I can't help but be down about the class who used to take care of me. There were a lot of nice little girls and boys in that class, and I haven't seen them in months, now. But if you gave me back, you would barely see me anymore, either. And even the kids in that class will move on to the next grade, soon. So, don't worry about it, that's just how life works."

Miranda had figured this was what her change in mood had been about. "I'm sorry, Mary. The school year's almost over, too. Is that why you've been even sadder lately?"

"That's exactly why," Mary replied. "Even if I hadn't run away, most of those kids would never see me again after the school year was over, except for a few of them who would visit me. I've been a school pet for a long time now, and I know that's how it goes. It's just how it goes."

After hearing how Mary really felt about it, Miranda knew that she had to stop being greedy and help her friend. She didn't know how she would manage it under her father's supervision, but she had to bring Mary back to her family.

"I'll do it," Miranda determined. "I'm going to take you back to Ms. Webb's class. I shouldn't have kept you to myself for this long in the first place. I'm really sorry. I didn't want to share you, and it was selfish."

Mary suddenly perked up. Everything about her demeanor seemed to change. "You would really do that for me? I can't believe it — that's so kind of you!"

Miranda looked down like Mary just had. "It's not, really. I should have done this a long time ago, from the very beginning, when I found out who you belonged to. You haven't even been happy here, anyway. It's my fault you went through all that in the first place." Miranda almost started to cry, but Mary stopped her.

"Don't say that. You're a young girl who is still learning things about life. I shouldn't have expected you to give away your new pet so soon," Mary said.

Miranda took some very deep breaths to calm herself down. "I hope you're not mad at me... I'm just worried that things won't be the same if I give you back."

"They won't be, sweetheart. I wish I could tell you that they would, but in my years going through this, I know how things go. I'll stay in the classroom, and you'll go on with your life. Just like old students, you might see me sometimes, but not as much as I would want. You'll feel guilty, and I'll miss you most of the time. But then the moments that I do see you will be very special. They make everything worth it," Mary said.

Miranda didn't want to believe any of the things her hamster was saying, but she just tried not to think about it. She told herself that she would see Mary every day.

"I have to talk to my daddy in the morning and tell him who you belong to," Miranda said. "I know I can't tell him you talk, so what am I supposed to do?"

Mary thought about telling Miranda to simply say she ran away, but she didn't want her to think that lying was OK, either. At this thought, she realized she didn't know what the little girl should do. Anything that she did to bring her back to the school would need her to lie, and Miranda was an impressionable little girl.

Mary was impressed when she was the one to think of an idea that didn't involve dishonesty. Miranda said that she would bring a photo of her hamster to school, making sure that Ms. Webb's class saw it, too. Then at least one kid would recognize Mary and beg her to take their pet back. After that, Miranda would be able to say honestly that she found out the hamster was the classroom's, and ask her dad to bring her back.

"I have a question," Miranda said all of a sudden. "I named you Mary, but since I didn't have you first, that means they called you something else. Why didn't you tell me your real name? And what is it?"

"In class, they call me Rose," she said. "But it's just a name, so I didn't want you to think you did something wrong by calling me something else. I like the name, Mary, too. You can keep calling me that."

"I will," Miranda said, smiling for the first time in the whole exchange.

"Go to bed now, Miranda," her hamster said. "You have a lot to do tomorrow, and I don't want you to be tired for school, either."

"Good night, Mary."

The two of them went to bed. In the morning, when she

went to school, Miranda did everything she was supposed to do, and there was one kid who said the photo was of his class's runaway hamster. She figured out it was Charlie, and remembered that she would have to tell on him when she took Mary back.

When she got home, Miranda was ready to do what she had been waiting to do all day. She dropped her backpack by the door and walked straight into her father's library. He was ready on his chair like he always did.

"Daddy," Miranda said. "I took a picture of Mary, and everyone at school was saying it was the class pet who ran away."

He slowly put down his book and took off his glasses. It seemed like he got very into the story he was reading and was taking a moment to reorient himself to what his daughter was saying.

"They really recognized their hamster? It sounds like they really liked her, then. But she did run away, Miranda," her father said. "I don't know that I want to trust kids to say when a hamster is theirs. Are you sure it was really their hamster?"

She wished that she could tell her father the truth about what Mary had told her, but she knew that Mary said that would frighten him, so she didn't.

"I am sure. They had a picture of her in that classroom, and she looks exactly the same as it. She has the same fur color, and she's the same size. Plus, everyone in that class swore to me that it was their old class pet," Miranda said.

"I'm sure they think it's their hamster, but that doesn't mean she is," her father said. "Either way, Mary is ours now, so don't let the other kids pressure you into taking her here."

Miranda went over to her room and told Mary what her dad said.

"I heard," Mary said. "It's okay. It sounds like there's nothing you can do about it, so just don't worry. I'll just be your pet. I'll feel better again, eventually."

Mary curled up into a ball and turned to the back corner of her cage. Miranda didn't think she looked like she felt better at all. But her dad said that she wasn't allowed to take the hamster back to her past owners. She was perplexed at what she should do.

She had an idea of what she should do, but she didn't want to sneak around her dad. Miranda knew that the school was opened early in the morning before she normally got there, and Ms. Webb was one of the teachers who was known to get there the earliest. If she got up early and took Mary with her, she could bring Mary back and tell the teacher what happened with Charlie.

When she thought about it, Miranda realized that there wasn't a way to do this while telling the complete truth. This was because even if she had her father's permission to return Mary, she wanted to tell the teacher about Charlie's treatment of the hamster as well.

She knew for a fact that this had happened because of what Mary told her, but she couldn't just say that the hamster had told her what Charlie did herself. That meant she had to tell Ms. Webb that she had seen what happened when this was not actually the case.

What Miranda did was tell herself that maybe sometimes, it is OK to tell a little fib if it meant it would protect someone. She wanted to protect Mary from Charlie, and she wanted to bring her back home, too. In order to do those two things, her only option was to tell a few small fibs.

The following morning, Miranda scooped up Mary in her hand and put her in the back pocket of her bookbag. She hadn't told her about her plan the night before, because she knew that Mary wouldn't approve of her lying to her father. But as smart as Mary was, she wouldn't be able to get out of her book bag when she zipped it, and she knew she was doing what was best for her.

Mary had been sulking in her cage the entire time since she got home from school the day before and told her that she didn't have her father's permission. Miranda thought she was probably secretly happy about what Mary was doing. But she wasn't able to admit it to her.

It was so early in the morning that it was barely even light outside because the sun had just come up. Miranda took the long mile-long walk to bring her hamster to the school. The entire trip, Mary pesters her to walk back home at once.

"Your dad didn't tell you that this was acceptable," Mary

kept saying. "I don't want you to get in trouble for this. Turn around this instant, Miranda. This isn't what you should be doing."

Miranda endured this for the whole long walk until she got to the school, and she needed help to figure out where the classroom was. Reluctantly, Mary told her which hallway it was in. It had been a long journey, but Mary was finally going back to her old owner. Ms. Webb was at her desk when Miranda entered.

Before speaking to the teacher, Miranda simply unzipped her backpack and took Mary out. She was extra careful with the hamster around Ms. Webb, much more careful than she had been when she was at home. She held her with both hands and slowly walked over to the cage that was still on the window, sill at the other side of the door.

"It's Rose!" Ms. Webb exclaimed. "I thought the children were out of their minds when they were saying Rose was still around. I assumed I would never see her ever again. Oh, my goodness! This is crazy!"

Miranda thought to herself that if she knew all the things she knew, it would be too crazy for her to handle. But she didn't tell her any of it, because of what Mary (now Rose) had told her: adults would be too scared to be able to handle knowing that an animal could talk.

She didn't say it directly, but Miranda did make some jokes about it for her former pet's sake.

"Rose is a very smart hamster, Ms. Webb," Miranda said. "One night, when I couldn't sleep, I walked out into my house's library, and Rose was reading a book under a lamplight."

Ms. Webb just laughed. "I'm sure that was a very strange thing to see."

"Then she told me that she learned how to read from your class," Miranda continued. She had realized that even though the hamster told her not to give away her secrets, it didn't really matter what she said to the adults, because they wouldn't think she was serious. Ms. Webb would simply laugh or smile at whatever claim Miranda made about her hamster.

But she didn't want to push things too far. She thought she owed the teacher a bit of an explanation. "I got her for my birthday. My daddy found her on the street and gave her to me as a present, but when I showed people pictures of her, they said it was Rose from this class. I called her Mary, but Rose is a very nice name, too," Miranda said. Before Ms. Webb could laugh again, Miranda took a deep breath and got ready to tell her little fib. "Oh, Ms. Webb, there's something very important I have to tell you. I didn't know it was the same hamster at the time, but before Rose ran away, I saw a student in your class treating her really meanly. He was poking at her with pencils."

"That must be why she ran away," Ms. Webb said seriously. "Thank you for telling me, Miranda. You're a very strong girl. You can be sure that she will be safe here from now on."

Mary walked about inside the cage. She didn't get settled right away, although Miranda could tell she was happy to be there. Mary faced Miranda, but saw that Ms. Webb was still there, so she didn't say anything.

"Ms. Webb, is it okay if I have a little time with Rose?" Miranda said. "I'm going to really miss her."

"Of course, you can! Let me go into the teacher's lounge

and get some work done in there," the teacher said. She picked up some books and papers and headed out of the room. Mary was free to talk again.

"It's not too late, Miranda," she said. "Part of me doesn't feel right about not being your hamster anymore. And your dad is going to be upset that I'm not there. You can tell him that I ran away, but you've already lied for me, and you're too young to be doing things like this."

"I can't keep you away from your family," Miranda said simply. "But don't worry about it. Maybe you're right that we won't see each other very much anymore, but you were so sad without the kids from this class, and I couldn't let that go on. I got you something, too."

Miranda pulled out the storybook that she found Mary reading the first night that she discovered her hamster could talk. With some effort, she hauled the heavy book out of her bag and put it outside the cage where she could read it, leaving it on the page she was last on.

"This is where your bookmark was," Miranda said. "I don't know if this is exactly right, though."

"It's perfect. I hope you do see me again soon," Mary

said sadly.

"Of course, I will. It won't even seem any different," Miranda promised. "I may not be in your class, but I'm going to see you all the time. I'll get you gifts, I'll read you stories, and when the teacher isn't looking, I'm going to take you out of the cage and we'll find new books for you in the school library."

"That sounds like a lot of fun," Mary said. "Thank you for being my owner, Miranda. I know that I wasn't that great to be around for the last couple of months, but you should know that I still loved having you around. It was just that I missed all those other kids too."

"I know that," Miranda said. She zipped up her bookbag. "Well, I have to run home now. If I don't hurry up, my daddy will notice that I'm not home. I don't want him to get worried."

"Yes, hurry home, Miranda," Mary said. "I'll see you soon."

Miranda ran home as fast as she could. Thankfully, he wasn't awake yet. She was really worried that he would wake up and notice that she wasn't home, but she knew that he was more of a night owl than an early bird, so she thought it was a reasonable risk to make.

Next came the part of the plan that Mary had just told her she didn't approve of. But she didn't approve of being taken back home either, and this was the only way for Miranda to explain the hamster being gone without her father knowing that she had gone to school by herself.

"Daddy!" she shouted. "Where's Mary? Do you know where Mary is?"

She ran to her father's door with an urgency as if her hamster really had run away. She heard him start to get up, but he took a long time to answer her cries, so she ran into his room anyway. He was scratching his eyes like he didn't know what to say.

"She's not in her cage?" he finally said when she stood at his bed.

"No, and I can't find her anywhere," she said.

Eventually, he got out of bed and helped her look for the hamster, even though Miranda knew they wouldn't find her.

"It sounds like she's the kind of hamster that likes to run away," her father said. "I wonder how many owners she's had before us. Maybe she really was that class pet you were talking about..."

"Maybe she was," Miranda said, trying to sound innocent.

"I couldn't find her anywhere, and neither could you. There are only so many places to look in this small house, so we may be out of luck, kid," her father said. "I'm sorry. You didn't even like any of your other birthday presents, did you?"

Miranda knew she had to seem upset, so she tried her best to act like it. "It's okay, daddy. Hamsters run away all the time. All the kids I know who had hamsters had them run away, too."

The two of them spent some time that morning watching cartoons before Miranda had to go back to school. The whole time, she was thinking about all the things she and Mary could do after she was done with class. Maybe no one would notice that she was gone once school was out. After all, the kids in the class only took care of her during the day, so she thought they probably wouldn't even notice if she was gone for a little while.

"Daddy, I want to play with my friend Rose after school," Miranda said.

"Rose? I've never met this friend of yours, but as long as you just play in the neighborhood, it's OK with me," her father said.

Miranda nodded and smiled. It looked like things wouldn't be so different after all.

Herman Hermit Crab gets Crabby

He swings and hits the baseball and it goes soaring way to the outfield. Herman Hermit crab scurries down the base line-safe at first. He high fives the base coach and gets ready to watch and see if he can steal 2nd base. The next batter gets up and gets ready to hit the ball. Swish- STRIKE 1

"Come on buddy!" yelled Herman "you can do it- hit that ball."

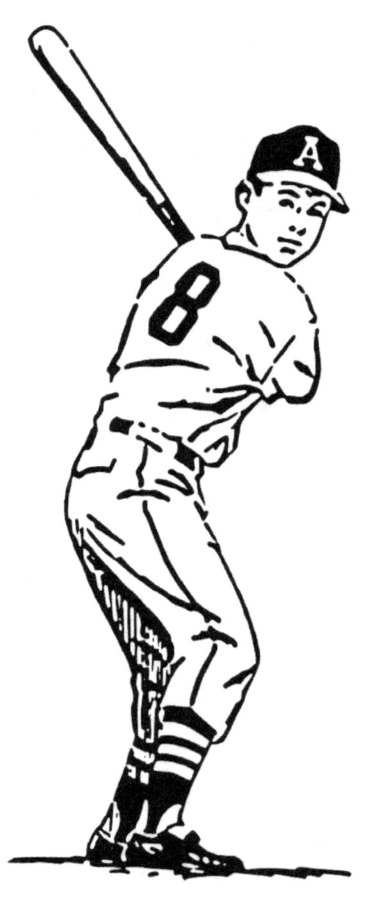

The pitcher winds up and throws the ball. Herman starts to run and steal 2nd base. The batter swings again- SWISH-Strike 2. But Herman made it to 2nd base. He began clapping his claws and cheering on the batter again, "You can do it- Hit me home!" Herman yells from

2[superscript]nd[/superscript] base.

Here comes the pitch and Herman starts to steal 3[superscript]rd[/superscript] base…. "FOUL BALL." Shouts the referee of the home plate. Herman scowls and heads back to 2[superscript]nd[/superscript] base.

Next 2 Pitches- "BALL" yells the umpire.

This is it Herman knew he could steal 3[superscript]rd[/superscript] on this next pitch so he crouched down and got ready to bolt down the baseline. The Pitcher winds up and lets the ball roar across the plate and Herman takes off. The catcher throws the ball but Herman slides in and is safe.

"HaHa I knew it," Herman said proudly "I knew I'd make it," he tells the 3[superscript]rd[/superscript] base coach.

The count is now 3 balls and 2 strikes; a full count. Herman watches the pitcher and looks at his coach for the sign to steal the base or wait. He gets the sign to wait. "Oh man, I could make it," Herman mumbles under his breath. He turns to his coach, "Let me steal home coach I can make it, I know I can."

"No wait here Herman, I think we can score if he hits the ball, if not we will wait for next batter." The coach encouraged Herman to wait. Herman made a grumpy face and stood on 3rd base kind of pouting. The batter swung and blooped it right down the third baseline. Herman wasn't paying attention, and he began to run. The 3rd base player picked up the ball tagged Herman and then threw it to first to get the batter out. A double play.

Herman stood there with a shocked look on his face. "Come on Herman lets go, we need to take the field," the coach said as he ran back to the dugout.

Herman walked back to the dugout very unhappy. He grabbed his mitt and headed out to the field. He walked out to center-field dragging his feet and taking his time.

"Batter up!" yelled the umpire. Herman was not even out to his position yet. He turned and scowled at the umpire as he made his way out to the outfield. Herman stood out there like he was waiting for a bus. He didn't move when a ball was hit and he didn't cheer on his team when they made a good play. Finally, they got 3 outs and Herman's team headed back in to bat.

"What's your problem, Herman?" Asked one of the

players.

"Hello-I got out. Didn't you see that?" Herman snapped with a crabby voice.

"We all get out sometimes; it's not a big deal. If the coach sent you and you got out it's not your fault you were doing what you were told to do." Another player chimed in.

"Well he DIDN'T send me but I knew I could make it," Herman grumbled.

Herman team made it through the batting order and Herman was up to bat again. "Herman, you're up!" His coach called out. Herman grabbed his bat and slumped his way to the batter box. Herman stood there waiting for the perfect pitch. He just watched as the pitcher pitched 3 strikes in a row. Herman was out. He dropped his bat and grumbled all the way back to the bench.

"Hey, your crabby attitude is not helping the team." The next batter said as he walked toward the plate.

"Whatever!" Herman snapped.

The inning was over and Herman's team was taking the field.

"Herman, I'd like you to sit this inning out. We are a team and everyone needs to participate to do well." His coach said.

Herman flopped down on the bench and watched as his team fielded ball an made outs.

"Herman, you are a good player...but you could be great," His coach said as they sat watching the other players. "You need to be a leader even if things don't go as you hoped. Your attitude affects everyone. If you stay positive the team can be positive or at some point, they just won't want to play with you."

Herman sat, listened and thought about what the coach had said but he was still crabby about getting out. But what the coach had said seemed like a good point. Even if Herman got out if he could try to learn from the parts of the game, he didn't like he could learn to be a better player and maybe teach other players tricky tricks to play better.

"Can I please go back in coach?" Herman asked the next

inning.

"I don't know Herman, how is your attitude?" Coach questioned.

"I am ready to do better. I understand that if I am crabby about what I did, it seems like I am crabby about what everyone does and I didn't mean for that to happen." Herman explained.

When the team took the field the next inning Herman ran out to his position and began being the team player, he knew he was. He was cheering on the team members who made plays and congratulated them when they made an out. Soon all the other players began to chime in on the team support. Herman stood in the outfield and felt proud that he was able to change his attitude and not be so crabby.

He realized that even when things don't go your way you can choose how to feel about it and choosing to look at the good things always makes you feel better.

Brother in Arms

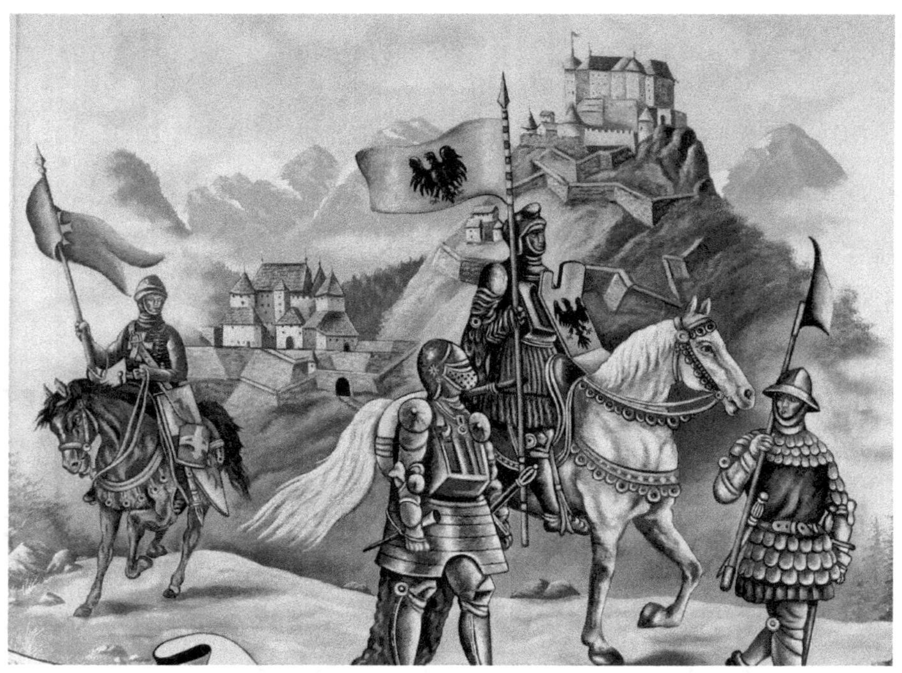

Calvin and Alexander were brothers who grew up together in the same castle. As teenagers, they are both squires to brothers, learning how to be knights. Calvin is a year older than Alexander but Alex is a fast learner and is working hard to become a knight as quickly as possible. They were both working to prove they would be good knights. They commissioned their own weapons and armor, they just needed to spend some time learning to fight well. Alexander is squire to Arthur. As a squire,

Alexander is learning to battle on and off his horse. He practices daily and shows his allegiance to the King. Calvin is squire to Clifford. He is learning to fight and which horses are best in different situations. They are both learning the same thing, how to be a knight. They help their knights get ready for battle. They are each waiting for the time they will go with their knights into battle. For now, they practice. Calvin and Alexander have not yet had to fight each other, but they know they will eventually meet on the practice field. Alexander is rising through the ranks quickly so they will be matched against each other soon.

One day, Calvin was training with the other squires, practicing the hand to hand fighting by beating another squire in a cruel manner. Alexander happened to see the fight and stepped in to stop the unnecessary beating. Alexander did not know, at first, that it was his brother who was beating up the helpless squire. When he noticed who he was disarming, he was amazed.

"Brother? Why are you so cruel to this young man? You are far bigger and far stronger. We are practicing. Why would you want to lame this boy for the rest of his life?", asked Alexander.

His question was answered with a sneer from Calvin, "I am showing what I can do. That way, no one has to guess if I will fight well. They can see for themselves that I can fight. I show everyone each day that I intend to fight to the death for my King."

"Well, this will not happen if you kill the King's men each day. You should be helping the squires who are not as good as you. The purpose of the practice is not to hurt your fellow squires. It is to learn how to behave in battle. You should not be so brutal when it is not necessary," responded Alexander.

Alexander could see that Calvin did not enjoy being reprimanded. His eyes started to narrow and he looked like he was squinting. Alexander knows this is a sign of anger. He smiled to try to soften the words that he already said, and tried to think of a way to get Calvin to smile back.

"Calvin, remember when we were little boys and you saved that injured bird. You nursed it back to health and set it free. That bird stayed around you for many years after. He would fly away, but he always came back a few days later to check on you."

"Why are you bringing up all this stupid kid stuff," asked Calvin. "I was young back then. That was a long time ago. You know that we are nearly men and I am here to show everyone that I will be a great man and a great knight. If you are not here for the same, get out of my way or I will beat you down as well."

Alexander did not know why his brother had changed so much, but he did not want to fight with him. He turned around and walked away.

Alexander was taught early in his training to always face the battle in front of you. He was taking a chance by turning his back on Calvin, but he could not bear to see his older brother changed to such a hard man. Yes, he agrees with Calvin. They are nearly men. There is a difference between them now and they may never be able to be the carefree boys they were. It did not make Alexander happy to realize it.

Calvin and Alexander continued to train to become knights by acting as squires. They learned about weapons. Calvin learned, but he did not take the same care with his knight's weapons as did Alexander. Alexander understands that weapons are a means to an end. They must be cared for carefully to be sure the metal is strong to strike and protect the knight. Protecting the knight protects the King and the kingdom. Arthur taught all this to Alexander and they both believed in the rightness of this idea. Calvin was taught to inspect the weapons. If Clifford did not like the looks of a weapon or shield, he discarded it. He had a stockpile of weapons he took from knights beaten in battle. Calvin was responsible for making sure the weapons and armor were in good shape and at the ready. Clifford was a valiant knight and had many battle victories. He killed many men and took whatever he could use or sell from the battlefield. It made Clifford rich and he shared his bounty with the King. The King showed his appreciation by inviting him to the castle and Clifford was invited to all the best festivities as a guest of the King. Because of this, Calvin learned that winning was the most important thing about being a knight. Clifford was very popular with the King and Calvin hoped to be as well.

To Arthur, a victory meant something different. Arthur

had won many battles as well, but he did not like killing men and boys barely out of their youth. He did what was necessary took no pleasure in it. Alexander could see that each death took a toll on Arthur but that is how battles work. It is Arthur's life and is Alexander's life. Alexander and Calvin fought for the same King to protect the land and property of the King and their own family. Calvin loved the battles and the King's celebrations. Alexander loved the kingdom and the thought that his family and others would be safe for another time.

The King hosted tournaments for the knights to practice and prove themselves worthy of being part of his feudal forces. The knights used the tourneys and an opportunity to teach the squires in a military situation, but not a deadly one. The squires used all the skills they were learning during the tournaments. Many squires were noticed by the King for good and for bad. As it happened, the King liked the money he gained from the knights like Clifford. They couldn't use everything found on the battlefield and if Clifford was willing to share the spoils with him, the better for the King. Arthur had a pesky habit of letting the losing knights pledge their allegiance to him and the King. Having a larger army was nice, but money is better. Every knight added was gold he did not receive. He would never tell either of the knights his preference, but he really did prefer to fill his coffers. The tournaments were a way to see if any of the knights Arthur brought into his fold we're good at what they did. Many were and they seemed to like being part of Arthur's inner group. Clifford had people around him who liked to have a good time and they liked the adventure of battle. In the King's mind, there is room for both types of knights.

One tournament day, it seemed that the knights of both Calvin and Alexander were both signed up to participate. The tournament will be held at a vast estate of a nobleman not many hours ride from the castle. It seemed likely that their family would be there to see all the sights. Calvin sent word that the two would be part of the tournament and he wanted to humiliate his brother in front of Father and mother. It will be the best gift Calvin could give himself. A display of strength and intelligence in front of his family, Clifford and the King will do a lot for his goal of knighthood. Defeating his brother will do the opposite for Alexander. Because Calvin was older, he had acquired more weapons and his armor was better fitted. Alexander was still growing and his armor would fit well one day and when he next went to put it on, it would be ill-fitting. But Alexander felt that Calvin was waiting for the opportunity to fight against his own little brother. Alexander had never been forgiven for breaking up the fight months earlier. Alexander was preparing for a long, exhausting tournament.

Calvin was very happy to have an opportunity to assist Clifford in his battle against the knights Arthur. Today would be the day that his brother would pay for daring to question the actions of his older brother. Calvin knows the noble art of knighthood and has been studying for longer. Calvin felt his brother was not only weak of body but weak of mind. He did not have what it takes to be a knight, from what Calvin could see. Calvin planned to conceal his attack during the melee. He felt sure he could take care of his brother and no one would be wiser. He was wearing the banner of his knight and saw that his brother was wearing the banner of his own liege. There will be lots of chaos as soon as the tourney starts and Calvin has plans to use the chaos to his advantage. He has a small knife he will use to cut the straps of Alexander's saddle. This will cause Alexander to fall off his horse in front of all the knights, the women, the noblemen, the peasants...everyone watching the tournament. His knight will probably dismiss Alexander as his squire. Calvin was happy. He wanted Alexander to be ruined.

Calvin saw a tunic with the coat-of-arms of Alexander's knight. He put it on over his own and made his way into the encampment of his enemy. Calvin had done this many times in times of battle so he moved easily among the knights and squires. Though Calvin did not notice, the camp noticed that the stranger moving in their midst. They were a close group and tended to know each other. A young squire was set to follow Calvin. He saw Calvin cutting the saddle straps on the horse normally used by Arthur's squire. He went back and reported what he saw to his knight. Arthur was informed and told Alexander to switch his saddle and get his own repaired. Alexander was angry that his brother tried to sabotage him in such an awful way. He was sure it was Calvin. He consulted with Arthur to see what he should do to end the feud with his brother. Alexander was not feuding, but Calvin was. Arthur suggested a long talk with Calvin to see if he is willing to stop the feud. Alexander set out to find his brother in the mob of people

When Alexander saw Calvin, he was with their family. They were all gathered together and looked happy to be together. Alex walked up and joined them all. They were happy that both their sons were safe.

Their mother walked to both of them and kissed the cheeks of each don. "Calvin, I'm so glad to let us know you would be near. We have missed you both so much."

Calvin just smiled. As he hugged his mother, Calvin looked over his shoulder and gave Alexander a sneaky smile. Alexander knew then that the feud would always be there for Calvin. He did not care if their dear mother and sister saw Alexander trampled by horses or lamed in the tournament. So, Alexander bid goodbye to the group and set off to ride next to his knight

He checked and rechecked all of his equipment and all of his weapons

He did the same for his knight. And they set off for the melee. It happened that Clifford and Arthur were marched in the joust. As part of the tournament, the squires would do a joust first. Calvin was sure he would knock Alexander off his horse easily because Calvin was sure Alexander was weak and he was sure Alexander's saddle was weak.

Before the joust, the two brothers met in the center of the list (the path the horses run along the rail) and Alexander surprised Calvin with angry words.

"Brother. You have held a grudge for many months. I was trying to you from your own anger an inability to control yourself. Now, I see that we will never be true brothers again. Go in peace. I am at peace with how we will be forevermore."

Calvin was a little confused as to why his brother was speaking to him of peace. But he would not let him have the last word.

"Brother. It doesn't matter what you thought you were doing. Have your peace. I will have riches. Do you see my fine suit of armor? It is the armor of a true warrior. Go to your post and prepare to fall. The peasants are waiting to see you fail." Alexander did not speak again he turned his horse and trotted away.

Calvin was sure of his victory over his brother. He had

made it so things would go his way. He looked at his brother who was seated proudly on his stallion. Calvin turned his horse around and suddenly, his horse bolted. Because of the armor, Calvin was not able to move easily and soon he found himself leaning off the horse and tumbling to the ground. His horse left the arena and headed back to the stable. There was laughter. Everyone was laughing at him. He felt his face go red with the heat of embarrassment. Calvin's helmet became dented in the fall and was damaged so much that they had to call the blacksmith to remove it. All the while, people walked past him and laughed. Because Calvin was wearing Clifford's coat of arms, Clifford was not pleased. He can le by and tore the tunic off of Calvin and told him to report to the page section from now on.

Calvin was humiliated. For a minute, as he was falling, Calvin thought maybe God was getting back at him for trying to bully Alexander. But after it was all over, Calvin decided to find the horse and see if Alexander had caused the problem. Unfortunately, when the horse was found, what Calvin found was a bee sting. It wasn't even an act of sabotage. A bee stung his horse in the snout. The stinger was still in the nostril and the swelling was immense. An insect destroyed his life. He sold his weapons and armor by the end of the day and took his horse with the swollen face and returned home with his family. There is no way he could be a page. He might as well become a monk. Yes. He would get back at Alexander. He will join the church and crusade against the knights. If Calvin can't be a knight, he doesn't want Alexander to be one either.

Chivalry Is Not Dead

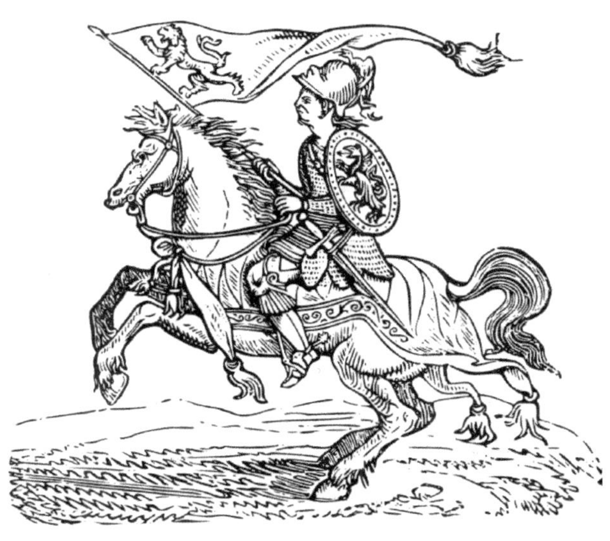

Alexander is a squire and has pledged his allegiance to the knight, Arthur. Alexander is working very hard to be dubbed a knight Arthur. He tries to be chivalrous at all times. He didn't realize how important the Code is, in life until recently. Alexander had a falling out with his brother. His brother was a squire for a knight who had a reputation for not exactly following the code of chivalry.

Alexander respects the code and wants to be sure when he is a knight, his fellow knights do the same. One day, when the band of knights was traveling across a pitted and scarred land they came across a village that seemed to be abandoned. One of the squires signaled that there was movement in the village. We were not sure if it was an animal or perhaps a squatter so some of the knights were sent to scout out the area. If nothing else, it would be a chance for the knights to rest. They had fought a long battle and were making their way back to their own lands. Their group was larger after the battle than before it. Though there were wounds that would need to heal, the loss of men was not as large as it could have been. Some of the defeated knights joined the ranks of Arthur's group. They pledged their loyalty to Arthur and his King.

The scouts came back with the news that there are families living in the ruins of the village. This did not change our plans to stop and rest. We entered the village and called all to come forward and stop hiding.

"Come forward, people. We are not here to harm. We simply seek a place to rest our tired bodies and water our horses," announced the herald as we made our way down the main road.

People began to peek out from behind the corners of the buildings that were still standing. Arthur dismounted from his horse. Alexander did the same and gathered the reins of both horses. Arthur walked out ahead of the group. He was heading for the building where there was movement. Everyone seemed to be waiting to see what would happen. None of the knights and squires were expecting what happened next.

Suddenly, there were rocks being launched from above towards Alexander and the group of knights. The band of fighters was able to use their shields to protect themselves from the barrage of stones. Arthur kept going forward and soon Alexander was by his side.

Alexander left the horses under the protection of another knight and joined Arthur at a quick pace towards the building. Just as suddenly as the barrage started, it ended.

Arthur announced his good intentions, "I don't think you understood what my herald announced. We just want to take a rest. Why do you attack us so cruelly?"

A voice answered from an old man walking towards the group, "We are a peaceful group. We do not have men here to protect us. They didn't mean any harm to you with the stones. Water your horses and then, please, keep going. There is nothing here for you to take. Whatever we had is already gone. Please, just leave us alone." Arthur and Alexander had never heard such a defeated plea.

"What has happened here," asked Arthur? Why are you all hiding? You must have chores to complete and work to do. Why is everyone hidden away?"

The old man had reached us now. He did not have a look of fear in his eyes. He looked as though he would accept whatever happened to him. His shoulders were slumped in his ragged shirt. He was clean but frail. If this is a security force for the town there is something very wrong. He offered greetings to everyone, looking Arthur in the eye, finally.

Arthur did not back away from the meekness in front of him, "Don't make me repeat myself, old man. What is going on here?"

The old man seemed to be offended at being called an old man. Alexander wondered at the bold way this man presented himself in the rags and frailty of defeat. He answered Arthur in a clear and booming voice, "We have been ravaged by men calling themselves The Knights of Clifford. The men of fighting age were struck down, our food stolen and our women...it was just cruel and the knights acted without honor."

Alexander was appalled. This was not the way knights are to act. Because of the Code of Chivalry, Arthur did not curse the actions of the knights who were here before, but he did not defend them either. It was too much to think about for Alexander but Arthur was not taken aback at all.

"You have no reason to trust us, but we are not like the other knights. We just want to get something to drink. Take a rest if you have beds. We have a coin. It is not our way to take what we want and move on. We have honor that seems to be missing from some of our kind."

The old man looked wary but signaled to have water brought out for the men. A young boy brought out a bucket with fresh water. The knights did not move to approach the water. The old man looked confused.

"Here is the water. What are you waiting for?"

Arthur answered without pause, "We are waiting for everyone to come out from hiding. We have already been attacked once.

The old man seemed to understand and signaled that it was okay for his village to show itself.

There were people coming from behind every pile of rubble, every tree and every doorway. But it wasn't a typical village of people. They were the very oldest and the very youngest except for the women. There were women of all ages. Everyone looked very thin and old. Even the children looked old. As Alexander looked at the people coming into the open area, he could have wept. He did not know how men of honor, knights who should be the most honorable of men, how could they leave the villagers to die a slow and anguished death.

"Where are your men," Arthur nearly shouted.

"I told you, they were killed. It was that Clifford. And they took all of our weapons and tools. They killed the blacksmith. We have been able to hunt with traps and bows and arrows but we haven't made anything big enough and sharp enough to use on anything bigger than a rabbit. We have many days when we have only a few meager vegetables to share, answered the old man.

He spoke for everyone and we could see everyone

nodding their heads in agreement.

The knights began to dismount after hearing the tale. Though everyone was tired and ready for a meal, it was apparent that there was no meal available. So, the knights began to unpack their travel provisions of dried meat, dried fruit, and hard bread. They made a pile between the villagers and the knights.

Arthur did not even have to turn around to know what his men were doing. He asked the villagers, "Who can turn this into the tastiest meal so that been may all eat a hot portion?" There was a rustling from the back of the group of villagers.

A girl no older than Alexander was pushed to the front and shyly spoke to Arthur, "I can cook. My family ran the inn. They are all dead except me. I know what to do."

"Good," answered Arthur. "Start on a meal."

A group of girls helped to gather everything in their aprons and they went to a building that had a sign hanging off its hinges that indicated it was, in fact, The Inn.

The knights passed around the water bucket and several boys brought more water. One of the older ladies showed the squires where they could take the horses for water and where they could munch on some grass and flowers.

The knights went along with the horses to try to wash away some of the dirt and sweat of the road and battle.

Arthur stopped to talk to a group of older men. Some had doubts about the integrity of the strangers. Others had hoped to be rescued. Alexander knew the knights would not leave without helping to put the town back together as well as they could and Arthur wanted to know what they needed most.

By the time it was worked out how the knights could help, the meal was ready and a plan was in Arthur's mind.

The village and the knights ate separately. The knights carried their meal to a field and ate noisily and happily. They had not had a hot meal in a few days and though it was not as hearty as they like, it tasted good.

The villagers gathered at the inn and ate well. They took small portions as they had grown used to eating very little. The taste, they were accustomed to. The portion of meat was not something they had eaten for months. They could feel the strength seeping back into their limbs by the time they finished.

As the villagers finished eating the knights were crowding the doorway. Alexander was elected to present the plans to the villagers. He started out shakily, his youth and inexperience showing in his red cheeks.

"Greetings villagers. Since we are here, we will help you with what you need to take care of yourselves."

As abruptly as Alexander started to talk, he finished and turned and left the building. The villagers thought him strange but began to clean up the tables in the inn. They needed to get back to the chores. They would have to try to check the traps and fetch more water. There were many things to do.

One of the knights set about the town looking for the smithy. He was used to caring for his shield and weapons and had some idea of how to make basic tools. He found the likely building, though the walls were no longer in existence. There was still a large hearth and workbench.

The knights had collected damaged and spare tools and

implements from the other knights. He was trying to get a good fire going in the hearth when he felt eyes upon him. They belonged to a pair of young boys. Both of them were smooth-faced and scrawny.

The older of the two, larger, anyway spoke, "Our family ran the smithy. Father was starting to teach us...." He broke off. He could not continue.

His brother moved towards the hearth and got to work getting the fire going. The brawny knight let him do it. As the boy made swift progress, the knight unloaded his pack of bits iron and leather. The boys watched and wondered, "Are you repairing your sword?"

"No. I'm going to make you a few tools so the fields can get planted and then harvested. I'm also thinking you need a good butcher knife and maybe a weapon. I think I can make something that's not too heavy so the ladies can handle them."

He was thinking the old men and boys could handle them too, but he didn't need to say it. Everyone still here feels something for not being able to stop the awful things that happened. The knights spent more than a fortnight in the village. With knights there to protect them, they were able to get the word to other villages close by that they needed a few things. Their situation did not seem as dire and they felt okay to have people in the village. The women were able to make some of the wares they were used to selling to neighboring villages and the knights helped to hire men from other areas to rebuild the village. Things were not perfect, but they were a lot better.

During all of this rebuilding, Alexander and Arthur had disappeared. Though the knights thought it strange, they knew the pair we're good men and waited for their return.

When the returned, no one was more surprised than the villagers. The two knights brought with them a huge wild boar and men that looked bedraggled and dirty and familiar.

"We brought some things you have been missing," said Arthur as the entered the new and improved village common.

Women and children of the village dropped whatever

they were doing and ran to the homely looking group. Some of their men had returned.

For some of the villagers, there was no happiness. They did not feel any worse than they felt that morning so no one was angry that only some of the men were able to return. Arthur and Alexander tracked the band of knights who attacked the village. They were able to find them only a few days ride away. It seems the band would stop every few days and pillage a town. This made their progress slow. They would gather men along the way. The men could either pledge their allegiance to Clifford and his Lord, or they would be taken along and used to work for the band of knights. They were not fed well so there were often among the group of slave labor. It took some time for Arthur and Alexander to return because they wanted to be sure the other slaves were able to get back to their homes as well.

One of the men, a farmer whose wife could not stop hugging him, explained further.

"We were trying to figure out, us that was stolen, how to get away so we could return home. We got in the habit of taking whatever we could from them that calls themselves knights after the slept from drinking too much ale. We got some knives and such. We had figured out how to unbind ourselves and everyone was freed for a short time each day. We took turns. We were working together to get away, those of us who didn't join up with those evil men. Sorry love," he said while looking at an angry woman with 7 or 8 angry kids around her, clinging to her skirts and scratching in the dirt. "Anyway," he continued, "One night we started hearing some strange noises out in the trees one. With one or two of us always unchained, we could look for food and such. Those knights did not bother to wonder if we were hungry. The two who were unchained went to see what the noise was. It was Arthur and Alexander. They were looking for us and now, here we are."

The long speech from the farmer told enough of the story for all to know how the men ended up back in the village. Of course, it wasn't easy to get away, but they did not want to worry the families with what happened to them. The villagers were all happy and the knights felt they had stayed long enough. They were ready to fight a new battle and so started to gather their belongings so they could move on. The villagers had enough meat to last for months. There were tools and weapons. Most importantly, the villagers had a willingness to work together and help each other.

Arthur went around the village to settle the debts. The band of knights had been staying at the inn and the stables. They ate food the villagers had been saving and some they got from neighboring villages. Arthur felt the village would need coin in the coming seasons, but he knew the coin would not be accepted. He was right. No one would accept the coin.

The innkeepers' daughter said it best, "If it wasn't for you, we wouldn't even be here."

Arthur went to the church and left the money on the altar. He was sure the coin would be put to good use. He was a good man and a good knight.

Garden Gnomes

Do you know what garden gnomes are? They are the cute little statues that you see sometimes 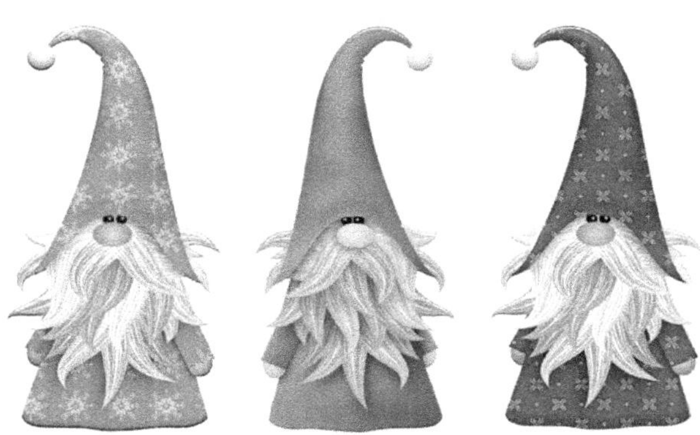 sitting outside on people's lawns and in their gardens.

Most garden gnomes have tall, pointy hats they wear and they are usually painted wearing brightly colored clothing that looks whimsical and fun. Have you ever wondered what it might be like to be able to paint your very own garden gnomes? What if I told you that you could paint your very own garden gnomes to put out in your garden right now, without having to move a single muscle? You really can- In your mind! Your mind is capable of doing many incredible things, including something called Visualization.

To begin your visualization practice, close your eyes. Really, close your eyes (unless you are the one reading this, of course!) To build a very strong visualization, it is usually helpful to first center yourself and be sure you are giving your brain the very best tools it needs to work with. In this case, that means oxygen, and oxygen means taking some good, deep breaths.

You are going to take some slow, deep breaths now, following along with my instruction: Breathe in very slowly, 1 – 2 – 3 – 4. Now breathe out, very slowly, 1 – 2 – 3 – 4. Excellent. Now again very slowly, 1 – 2 – 3 – 4 and breathe back out very slowly, 1 – 2 – 3 – 4 very nice. Once more very slowly in 1 – 2 – 3 – 4 and back out very slowly, 1 – 2 – 3 – 4. Great!

Take a moment to review how you feel. Are you comfy and feeling good? Okay, great.

Picture yourself, in your mind's eye, outside on a beautiful spring day. The sky is a pale blue above you and the sun is warming you where you sit. You have an artist's workspace set up with a wooden table that is about the same height as your waist, stocked with paints and paintbrushes of every color and every size. There are also several garden gnome statues beside the table, all the same light gray color of unpainted pottery.

You take a long, deep breath in and notice how fresh and clean the spring air is and you think to yourself that today is a spectacular day to be outside doing a lovely paint project. You look down and notice that you have on a long, black apron. Perfect! Now you won't have to worry about getting paint on your clothes.

You lean down to inspect the garden gnomes. Each one is unique and different. Some are smiling and others are making funny faces. Some are standing with their hands on their hips and some are crouched down petting a bunny rabbit or holding a little frog. There is even a garden gnome that is picking his nose!!! You laugh a little at this, gross!

That's when you see it: the perfect garden gnome for you! This garden gnome is wearing the typical pointy gnome hat but with a twist: it has a super-wide brim, like a sun hat and his hands are up in the air with his fingers outstretched like he is at a party or something! You know it will be so fun to paint and decorate this little guy.

You lifted the fun party garden gnome up and set him on the table. You take a couple of steps back, wondering what color you should paint his hat. You pull a paint palette out and inspect the color options: there is a light aqua blue, tangerine orange, bright cherry red, pale buttercream yellow, and a sparkly midnight black color. So many awesome choices, but you think that this little gnome needs a fun party hat, so you decide to start with the bright cherry red!

You look at the many paintbrushes available and decide that the hat needs one that is a decent size, so you pick up a paintbrush that is about as wide as a quarter. You dip it into the cherry red, swirling the color on to the paintbrush. You begin to paint the awesome party hat and smile as you watch the vivid cherry red slowly cover the entire hat.

Now it's time to move on to the garden gnome's outfit. Hmm. You look at your palette and decide that sparkly midnight black color would be the perfect color for the shirt, so you choose another wide paintbrush and dip it into the midnight black color, loving how sparkly it is! You begin to paint the gnome's shirt, watching in awe as the sparkly midnight black seems to glitter more and more with every stroke of your paintbrush. You love it!

The next step is to paint the little shorts, and you think

that the tangerine orange would be perfect, so you select another paintbrush and begin to paint the gnome's shorts a beautiful tangerine orange. You think that the tangerine orange is such an awesome color, you will keep the same paintbrush and just dip it right into the pale buttercream yellow to create a deep yellow-orange for the gnome's little shoes.

Now that you've painted your garden gnome's clothes, you step back from the table to look him over. His cherry-red hat, his sparkly midnight black shirt, tangerine orange shorts, and yellow-orange shoes are absolutely perfect! He is colorful and bright and looks like the perfect addition to your garden. You look over at all the other garden gnomes waiting to be painted and are very thankful that you get to paint all these cute garden gnomes. Next gnome is the one picking his nose!

You do not have to leave your garden gnomes just yet if you don't want to. You can spend as long as you want here and you can come back anytime you'd like.

You can create anything you want in your mind. Imagine where you want to go and build the picture in your mind. Be sure to imagine how you want it to smell, taste, hear and feel. The more detailed you can make your mental picture, the more you will enjoy being there.

It is all up to you. Perhaps as you drift off to sleep, you may find yourself back here with your paints and your garden gnomes, enjoying this beautiful spring day.

Topher's Ultimatum

Topher worked at an ordinary software company. When people asked what his job was, he just told 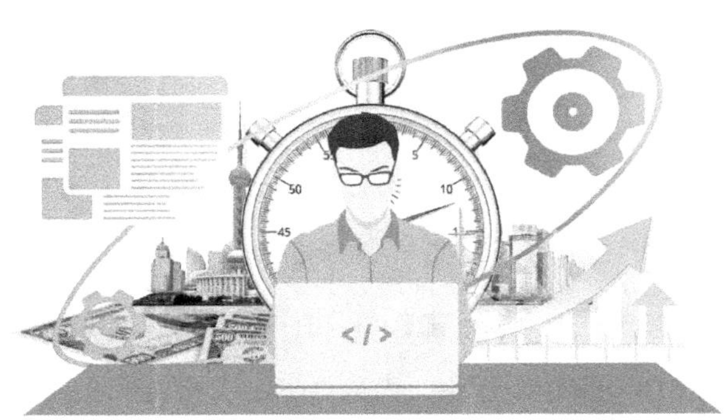 them debugging. If they were interested, he could tell them more about the intricacies of what he did, but no one ever was. Even he wasn't.

Not that he had many qualms with his life. He would often say that things being boring was a sign that he was lucky. It meant that he didn't spend his days fretting over big problems.

He spent his days dealing with very small first-world problems: the slightly more interesting to describe his job was to say that he fixed issues that people had with their cell phone software. He was one of the people who fixed the code behind what makes everyone's personal devices work. Again, he had no complaints about the life he lives being mostly uneventful. Topher didn't mind it at all, but there was one thing that made it worse, and it had to do with his boss, Sam.

He knew it was common for a person to hate their boss, but when Topher talked about how much he hated Sam, he didn't think they understood the gravity of his hatred. The reason he hated him so much was that even though Sam didn't do a much different job, he was paid significantly more.

What was more, Sam always seemed to be flaunting the nice things he could afford with his salary. If Sam didn't have a family, it would be different, but he knew that he did, so watching Sam's Corvette rolling into the parking lot every morning nearly drove him mad.

Topher had a family too: a wife named Wendy and two boys. He was paid relatively well, all things considered. But after everything was paid for as far as bills, he always seemed to be broke. Retirement seemed like a joke at this point. If there was an unexpected medical expense coming in the future, he wasn't sure how he would cover it. He knew for a fact that the insurance that Sam had for his family was much better, because he accidentally stumbled upon these records when doing normal work one day.

The thought of that accident gave Topher an idea, though. It was possible that there was something unsavory in the more detailed financial reports deep in the records that no one read. It was a long shot, but perhaps if he took a look, there would be something that he could use against him.

Topher felt vindicated when he found what he was looking for. He didn't find it in the financial records for Sam, but for the company. When he added up all the accounts receivable and compared them with the accounts payable, there was a huge discrepancy. Why did the company systematically end up with tens of thousands of dollars every week on the whole? There had to be something here that no one else was paying attention to.

Since they worked for such a big, powerful company, he could see how something like this could go unnoticed. But that didn't mean that corporate would be able to ignore it if it was brought to their attention. Topher couldn't say for sure if Sam was the reason for the discrepancy, but no one else could control the money that went in and out more than he could. He didn't really have to prove that he did it in the papers as long as he was scared enough of the accusation. Sure, there would be some consequences if he was wrong, but Topher was a programmer. He could always work somewhere else.

And he didn't think he was wrong. It made everything made sense. Sam's salary was significantly higher than Topher's, but with him having the pay the same expenses for having a family as he did, it just didn't make sense for him to have so much more extra money all the time. The missing money from the company accounts would explain it completely.

Now, he didn't really want to just rat Sam out. He could get no benefit out of that. What he wanted was some power that he would be able to attain if his hunch was right, and his findings would put Sam in jeopardy. Topher didn't want to be the boss himself; he was fine with staying in the position he was now. But he thought if Sam knew that Topher knew what he was doing, there was a lot he would be able to get away with that he wouldn't otherwise. His life had gotten stale, and this could lead to something new. And he hated his boss. He was killing two birds with one stone.

It wasn't that Topher wanted a promotion or a raise. It was that he was sick of being overlooked for these things. He told Sam as much when went to his office and made a deal with him.

Topher dressed noticeably differently that day. Even the men took a second look at him when he passed by. He was wearing a suit in place of his normal button-up and khakis. Only Sam, the boss, would ever wear a suit. But Topher was wearing a suit to send a message: a message that he would be the boss from now on.

He didn't make a meeting with Sam beforehand. He planned to do this on a Monday morning, just after he arrived. Sam always arrived at the building around 6, while Topher always got there around 8. This meant Sam would feel like he was settling into his weekly routine when Topher would suddenly come into his office and slam the stack of accounting papers on his desk.

Sam didn't say anything at first. He seemed absolutely confused as to what this would be about. But seeing the look on his usually non-threatening employee's face let him in on what was happening.

Still, Sam flipped through the pages first. Topher didn't say anything, because he thought the documents should speak for themselves. He also thought that on the off chance he was wrong, he could say that he saw a clerical mistake in the funds. But he really didn't think that was what was going on here.

Just as Topher expected, Sam didn't deny it. He came out with it pretty quickly.

"So, you started to read about what we really do around here," he said. "Shut the door, please."

Topher did. The two of them sat on either end of Sam's desk, quiet for a long while. Topher knew what he wanted, but he thought it was smart to see if Sam would have anything else incriminating to say first. This might go even deeper than he originally assumed.

Sam didn't say anything else, though. Not wanting to lose his moment, Topher finally spoke up. "What 'we' do around here? Your name might not be on this directly, but your signature is all over the code. This wasn't written by anyone else. I don't think this has to do with anyone else besides yourself."

"I meant that I'm not the only one who's doing this, Topher," Sam said. "Look, I understand where you're coming from. I used to be a moral person like yourself. But when I talk to my boss — the one who really ones this place — I start to see things more clearly. No, you're not the one in control here. Do you think I am? I most certainly am not. The ones in control here are the ones who own the damn place. I don't own any significant portion of the company — just the small piece that legally has to own. That's it. I don't control any of this," Sam said. "And the money — do you think they're missing it? Of course, they aren't. What thousands are to them are what coins are to us. They don't even notice it leaving our accounts. It's hard to believe for people like you and me, but it's true."

"People like you and me," Topher scoffed. "I know how much you make. And now I know how much you really make."

"Trust me, pal. If you really knew how much a billion dollars was worth, you would understand that you and I are truly in the same class. To the guys at the top, we're insignificant. Nothing that we do really affects their bottom line. All we do is our small parts in making their machines operate. That's it."

Topher noticed that Sam was chewing gum, which made him mad. He was already dominating the conversation, even though he was the one who should be. Sitting in there with just him made him pretty nervous if he was being honest with himself. Come to think of it; he thought this had to be the first time they had a one-on-one conversation. Every other time they had talked, it was in the presence of many more ears. But with the door secured shut right now, there was no way anyone was hearing anything they were saying.

"You misunderstood me when you said I'm being a moralist," Topher said. "I'm smart enough to know I don't have anything to gain from turning this in. I wouldn't get money or a trophy. You would just get in legal trouble, and I would probably have to show up in court. I don't want that at all."

"Let me make a wild guess, then," Sam said, sounding bored. "You're threatening to show this to someone if I don't give you a cut."

"Exactly right," Topher said. He was perplexed. Somehow, everything seemed to be going the way it was supposed to and wrong at the same time. He thought he wished that Sam had acted surprised at his finding or something. Instead, it was almost like he had been waiting for this to happen all along.

"I don't mean to take away all the excitement, buddy, but as you saw in our papers, it is all right there," Sam said. "Anyone who bothered to read what the code actually said, rather than just performing the operations, would be able to see that I was stealing. To me, this is the perfect crime. Who gets hurt? Do you really call some billionaires getting thousands less of their shares injustice? And if and when someone did find out, as you did, what would happen? I figured they would just want a piece of it, which you did. As far as I'm concerned, there's no harm done here. Obviously, I would have liked it more if I kept all of the money, but I don't need every penny of it if I'm being truthful. It's much more than I can spend or plan with. The fact that there are people out there with more money than this is pretty insane if you ask me. What are they doing with it? Just holding it?"

"You're getting a little political, Sam," Topher said.

"Whatever you say," Sam said. "I thought we were just chatting. Well, I suppose that does it, then. I know your bank. I'll start wiring half of it to you as the price of your silence. Does that sound all right with you?"

"It does," Topher said. He had already given up on having a big moment. He had thought for a bit that this would be about more than the money, and it was disappointing to see that at the end of the day, this really was just about money — which made it all seem like a typical part of his typical life.

The other reason for revealing these papers to his boss was to make Sam uncomfortable since he had harbored this resentment against him for so long. But now that he knew he could have found out this secret a long time ago and gotten a cut, he didn't feel like he made Sam feel on edge at all. If anything, Sam just made him feel like an idiot.

Topher didn't know how to react to all this. Somehow, even with how his life would surely change from this new influx of funds, he felt like he didn't get what he wanted out of this ultimatum at all.

He went home and gave Wendy the reason he had rehearsed for why they were about to have much more money than they used to: he had gotten promoted to Project Manager at the company. Wendy had never shown any genuine interest in his job, so she simply pretended to be proud of his accomplishment, but in truth, Topher had never cared about being promoted, either.

He didn't want to have more responsibilities than he already had, and he didn't get a power rush out of leading people as some people did. He only told Wendy about the promotion because it felt good, and because he needed some sort of rationale for all the things, he was going to buy with all his new cash.

Topher knew Wendy would tell him he was going overboard with the raise, but that was part of the fun of it all. He didn't want to worry about money anymore now that he was getting more than he knew to do with. His idea of luxury was buying a new hybrid vehicle, the newest gadgets; he started investing in new products based on their promise rather than the market history.

He could tell his family was much happier with money, too. Everyone who said that money couldn't buy happiness must have just never had it, because although the happiness he earned from it was fleeting in a way that he could tell, it was very much real happiness. His sons got their own credit cards, because he thought, why not? Now, he could afford it.

Contrary to the homemaker stereotype, Wendy did not actually spend money much differently than she used to before his promotion. Instead, she complained to him about how he was teaching their children bad habits. She said it was almost better before, because at least then they had a limit they had to stay inside. When they didn't have these limits, they became something she didn't recognize.

To Topher's dismay, the second person to express such concerns was his boss. Just as Topher had come into Sam's office that Monday morning, Sam went into Topher's cubicle. But instead of slamming down a stack of papers on his desk, he just started talking.

"Are you out of your mind, Topher?" Sam said. He kept his voice slightly down, but everyone was gone at the moment to eat lunch, so no one could hear them. "You can't have a closed-door meeting with me one week and then drive to work in an electric car the next. It looks very suspicious. I thought you had to be smart in order to notice the discrepancy in the account papers. But instead, it seems like having just a little bit more money has completely gone to your head. Did you even find the discrepancy because you were reading it normally, or were you just trying to find something against me? Because I'm starting to think the latter."

"People don't know what investments I'm making. Maybe I took out a loan for the car," Topher suggested. He was indignant that his boss continued to act this way, dragging out the feeling of dissatisfaction he had had when he showed him the paper in the first place.

"No one takes out a loan out of the blue like that, and if you were making investments that good, you wouldn't be here," Sam said. Topher hated how he always acted like he knew everything. "And you know you have to have money in the first place to make investments that pay off that much. Just think a little bit, please. You really need to settle down with all the spending. People might start asking questions. Every employee's pay is public, so we can all see that I didn't give you a raise."

Topher desperately wanted to catch Sam off guard, just once. "I could let the truth out at any time. So, what if I'm implicated? I was pressured by you. You wouldn't let me tell the truth. You intimidated me. I didn't think I had another choice."

Sam looked at him, expressionless. "You really don't think. What kind of crap do you think people really believe? Not that, I'll tell you. You don't get to play the victim in this; it won't work out for you. Though I have to admit, you would make for quite a convincing one, with how dim-witted you've been acting. It's hard to believe you're the one who threatened me. On what grounds do you stand on now, anyway? You are just as complicit in this as I am. No one is going to believe that you were threatened into having more money than you had before. No one."

"What do you want from me? I'm the one who discovered your secret," Topher said. "I would play nicer with me if

I were you."

Sam sighed. "Sure, I will, Topher. I am just trying to help us the best I can since both of our names are on this. There's no going back for either of us, so it's in our best interest to keep this as clean as possible."

Topher was tired of being treated like this. He was the one who could uncover Sam's secret any time he wanted, yet he treated being treated like some kind of idiot. "I have an addendum to add to our agreement, boss," Topher said. He grabbed his laptop case and started stuffing his things inside of it. "I don't want to come in here anymore. If you need me for someone, you can send me a call. Or an email. Better yet, don't try to reach me at all. I'm done coming into this place. With what I know, I don't have to anymore."

Sam didn't skip a beat. It infuriated Topher even further, but it didn't matter. He was already walking out of the building. "It's for the best, probably. The longer you stay here, the more questions people are going to ask. You won't even need a title here anymore. You'll have all the money you ever needed sent into your account."

"When you put it that way, this is the arrangement I should have asked for in the first place," Topher said. He went on his way home.

Topher's peace from quitting didn't last long. Even just hours after getting home, he started to get paranoid. He didn't answer calls or emails. He didn't know if his former boss had even tried to reach him, because if he did, Topher certainly hadn't answered them. The way he tried to keep his sanity was rocking back and forth, trying his very best not to check any of the ways he could be contacted.

He knew he should try to think about something else, but he became obsessed with it, and it didn't seem possible to do anything but stare at his blank computer screen without opening the email application.

The amounts he was receiving were astronomical right now, but he started to get worried about how things could change. Was it really as much as it seemed in the beginning? Would it cover his sons' college tuition now that he didn't earn a salary from his regular job any longer? Would he have to sell his electric car? The thoughts didn't stop racing through his head, and he felt like this had to be the last straw. Without reading any messages or voicemails that may have already been sent to him, Topher sent Sam an email saying that he was cutting all ties with the company: he didn't want to be contacted by anyone from there ever again. All he wanted was what he already had set up. He didn't say what he meant directly since email was a traceable mode of communication, but he figured Sam knew what he was talking about.

In other words, he still expected his cut to come virtually into his account. He had things to pay for, and knowing how devious Sam could be, Topher had a bad feeling he wouldn't be able to work at any other tech company after this. Sam had probably put Topher on a blacklist that would prevent him from getting hired anywhere else. This was the end of the road for his real career. His only choice now was to leave.

He discussed it with his wife in a different way than he truly saw it, but they were moving out of the country. After thinking of all the different places, they could go, he eventually landed in Granada, Spain. He thought they would probably not be bothered there. After just a month of preparations, he, Wendy, and their two sons flew over to their new home in Spain.

Spain had never been at the top of his mind before, but he chose it now because he was not willing to go anywhere where he could understand the language around him. Not now, when his paranoid was getting so out of hand that a few simple words in the next room might drive him berserk. As long as the people around him were speaking in Spanish, he didn't worry about things like this.

Of all the places they looked at online, Granda seemed like the most beautiful. There were many areas they could visit as tourists, but it was also a friendly place for foreigners without too much English being spoken there. They could expect many people to be able to understand them so they could take care of their errands without any issues, but English was not so common as to trigger Topher's paranoia.

Of course, Wendy did not know about this problem at all. As far as she knew, he was continuing to work remotely. She had no idea all of their money was coming from the illegal deposits he was getting through Sam.

Things were looking up after the move, mostly because it greatly helped him not look at his modes of communication for a short while. But when he did, he noticed something very disturbing. When he checked his bank account, he had stopped receiving half of the cut from Sam. From what he saw, he was getting the full 50%. On the surface, this was a good thing, but he had a bad feeling about this. He knew that Sam had to be setting him up.

But Topher didn't know what he could do about it. Sam stopped answering all of his calls. He figured this had to be his fault because this is what Topher asked him to do. But now, he didn't even have a way to confirm what was going on.

Then a month passed, and his worst fear was realized. He did not get the deposit on the day he was supposed to. His paranoia went to extreme levels at this point. Then, a day passed, and another day. The most still didn't come.

Topher knew what he had to do. He had to make his withdrawals before his bank was totally frozen. He wasn't able to withdraw all of it at once, but he was pleased to find out he could get most of it in euros.

It seemed like Spain was a very cash-friendly place, so he hardly had any problems with this at all. It was not all of the money that he would need throughout his whole life, but it was more than enough for the next couple years while he figured out what he and his family should do next.

He didn't hear back from Sam for two years. When he did, it was nothing good. He and Sam had a short conversation about what happened and what Topher should do. Topher was right: knowing that him moving away suddenly seemed suspicious, Sam started sending all of the money to him, instead of just the 50 percent. Then Sam sent this information to the corporate office, who had no choice but to send it to the authorities, or else they could get into trouble themselves.

If Topher ever went back to America, he would be in deep trouble. He knew it; his paranoia had been affirmed to be unclouded judgment. Topher hadn't been crazy at all to think they had to leave. If he wasn't in Spain right now, he would probably be in jail. Now he, Wendy, and the kids had no choice but to find a new life here in Granada.

He didn't know what came next for them, but he did know that it couldn't be in his home country.

Topher started working under the table for a bar, and even picked up some Spanish as he did it. The money wasn't nearly enough to pay for his sons' eventual college tuition or for his and his wife's retirement, but at least he felt like he was doing something about the problem.

He even started to sincerely enjoy the job. He had never worked with his hands before and made real, physical things. As a programmer and a software developer, he had only typed to create code that made pixels, which could technically be counted as physical things, but it was not at all the same.

Topher started to find a sort of happiness in doing this work. But things took a turn when Wendy came to the bar and saw him there. It looked like she had only gone in there for a drink — she did not expect to find her husband behind the counter at all. He hadn't expected to see her either, so he didn't know what to do or say when they saw each other. She demanded to know what was going on. Topher told her the truth, knowing that by now, there was no coming back from it. He had lost the job a long time ago, and he had even lost the large illegal deposits that had been sustaining them thus far. They still had plenty of money for basics, but there was no money for the future.

He could tell that this wasn't the first bar Wendy had gone to that night. The way she reacted broke him, but it didn't surprise him, because he knew how many mistakes he had made. Wendy walked out on him on the spot.

Topher didn't know if his family would be home when he got back, but he had a bad feeling that they wouldn't be.

When he got off his shift, he came home, and indeed his family was no longer there. They left no note, and the only traces of them that were left were the Spanish learning books that none of them had ever really mastered.

He sat on his bed and thought about how things could have gone differently. All of the money that they got for a short while was not worth all of this. He had lost everything: the money, his wife, his kids. He could have kept doing his normal job; he could have left the financial records alone, and just minded his own business.

It wasn't right that Sam got away with all this. He had a glimpse of hope, thinking that he could prove what Sam did, too. Then he thought back to what Sam had said: no one would believe him. And he was right. It was apparent that Topher had done wrong. He had even moved out of the country.

Meanwhile, Sam was already richer than everyone else in the office before Topher made all these mistakes. It was far more suspicious for Topher to be doing the things he was doing compared to Sam. He should have known that he couldn't get away with the same things.

But it was too late. The realization struck him so hard that he didn't know how to react to it emotionally. He was simply despondent. But not completely.

He had become a bartender in Spain. He had participated in a fraud that made him very rich for a period of time. He may have never been able to push any of Sam's buttons, but at least his life had seen some excitement. It wasn't much of a comfort, but when he looked back on it, he had taken these chances so that he could have stories to tell. And now he did.

The Love in Fire

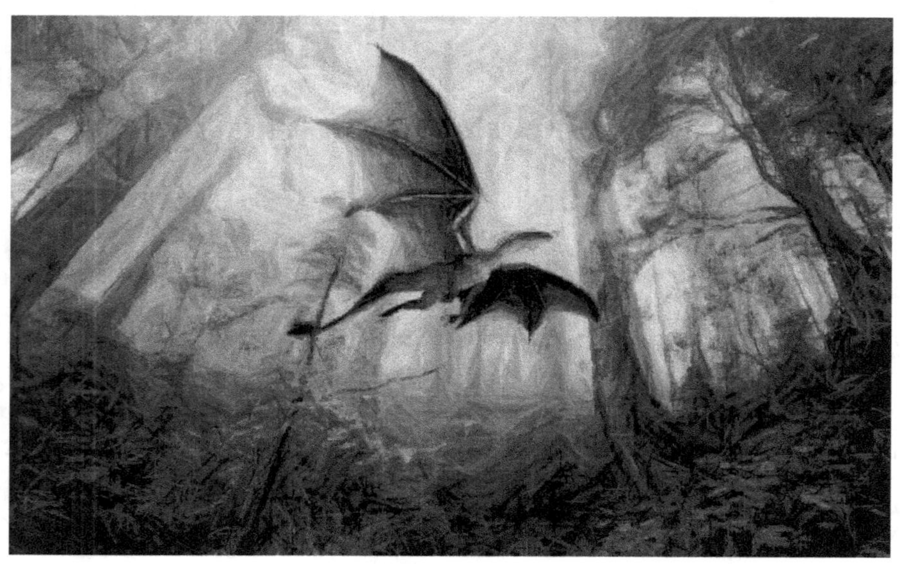

There was once a young dragon named Romulus, who roamed Whimsy hundreds of years ago. His family and friends referred to him as Rom. His scales were the color of slate with sharp white teeth that could frighten even the most seasoned warrior. His eyes blazed brilliantly, the essence of lava. Rom had an enormous wingspan with sharp boney protrusions at the tip of each. His tale was exceptionally long at fifteen feet, and he could wrap it around his body. The horizontal plated scales on his chest shone golden in the light of day. Rom was a rather regal looking dragon, poised enough to look both elegant and terrifying. Strangers always noted his eerie beauty as his breastbone puffed out in front of him, like a lion's mane.

Should you ever met Rom, you might initially be scared out of your mind. Getting to know the young dragon is another beast altogether. He was not the most graceful creature to ever sail the skies of Whimsy, frequently becoming distracted and running into trees. He was lucky that dragons have such hard heads.

Rom was also not possessed of the same fierceness that was commonplace among his species. He loved getting to know other creatures and spent his days watching the various beings of Whimsy from above. He was a loving and curious dragon, with a taste for adventure. Any other dragon that he's ever met just loved to fight. They were a ruthless species that often found their use in being contracted by villages for protection from enemies that mortals would not be able to guard against.

Dragons were not cruel or uncaring; it was just in their nature to spar. They would never just terrorize others for sport, but should they be tasked with protecting a town...they would enjoy the battle. All except for Rom that is. He was hardly ever around to be involved in these great wars. He could be found in the forest, making friends with any creature that was not immediately terrified by the way that he looked.

The young dragon was especially fond of elves. He found them to be lovely and mysterious. The elven race in Whimsy was tall and pale, with their skin reflecting a pale blue. Hair like the night sky fell around them, usually to their waists. They were a wise species that also valued learned and knowledge above everything else, not dissimilar to Rom himself.

Rom's most favorite elf was also his best friend, whom he referred to as Blue. Elven words are some of the most difficult to pronounce, so they were often given nicknames by those they meet. The race has a distinctly different vocal cord arrangement, making their mother tongue very trying for strangers. Luckily, they were all educated and fluent in the various other languages of the realm.

Blue was one of the first creatures that Rom had ever met who did not immediately flee from the sight of the imposingly statured dragon. The two shared many of the same interests and loved going on adventures together. They crafted a very special saddle that allowed the young elf to safely ride atop of Rom as he flew to their next destination.

One cold and dreary day, the pair decided that they would venture out in search of a tropical environment. Both had heard tales of a beach with pristine white sand contrasting against the vivid azure of rolling ocean tides. This was a land far south, where it was rumored to be warm all year round. Exotic species supposedly peppered the land, which made both Rom and Blue very eager to set sail. They treasured the relationships they formed with new beings.

They had no concept of how important their adventures were for connecting the various creatures of Whimsy. Rom specifically had broken many harmful dragon stereotypes that others hold about the race until they met him. Blue served as the diplomat in their operation, and he was responsible for establishing the first contact. Elves were much more approachable, which allowed him a chance to explain the kind nature of his scary-looking best friend. The pair bundled the young elf up because the frigid air would be almost unbearable for Blue as they cut through the cold rain at lightning-fast speeds. He would fashion a cocoon of sorts that they would stabilize around the saddle with ropes. They used thin pieces of wood to structure the mass. Large leaves would encompass the mass of fabric to repel the precipitation that they would encounter. A tube of steel would run from inside this cloth cave, to the outside air, so that Blue would not feel as though he was suffocating under the weight of his protection. The two were quite inventive about preparing for their travels and would do their best to anticipate obstacles ahead of time, mostly with the intent of keeping Blue safe. Dragons were fairly durable in comparison to elves.

Rom took to the sky with his passenger hunkered down and warmed on his back. The trip was made slightly more difficult with the added weight, but the young dragon was strong enough to keep flying. Hours passed, and it seemed to the pair like the coast might be a myth. They'd never been this far away from their stomping grounds before. As Rom passed a large canyon carved into the countryside, a man seated atop a cliff waved at him. He waved back before realizing that this man was far larger than a man should be. Rom felt his heartbeat sped up; he had just met his first giant! He could not wait to relay the experience to Blue!

Finally, night began to fall as Rom was beginning to lose some of his energy. He wished that he would have told his family where he was going; he just never dreamed that it would be so far away. The climate was getting warmer, but there was no ocean in sight. He hoped that his parents weren't too worried about him.

The pair stopped for the night, finding shelter in a forest. The trees were all very strange looking with rust-colored bark. They seemed to be spaced even distances away from one another, lending a very clean look to the woodland. They seemed to be swaying back and forth to a gentle wind. Blue swore that he heard the trees whispering to one another.

Rom and Blue had a serious talk about if they should continue onward or return home. They knew that eventually, their families would grow concerned about them, but they also didn't want to have wasted all the time and effort that their journey had taken thus far. They came to the conclusion that they would press on for now. They two set by a fire that Rom had created eating an elven herbal soup that Blue made from the plants around them and some dried meat that the two had packed for the journey. They laughed and told stories late into the night.

In the morning, Rom hunted down a cave where he would hide their cocoon contraption until they were on their way back. The climate was more like spring and less like the oppressive winter from back home. They set off once again to find their ocean, refusing to lose hope.

Again, the pair spent hours in the sky, watching the midday sun travel across the horizon and dip below. There was a stillness in the night air, as the two decided to continue their trip through the darkness. Rom was encouraged by a strange smell that hung thick around them. It was a saltiness that he had never experienced before. He harkened back to the rumors of the mysterious sea, as it was said to be filled with a briny water solution. The moon dusted a pale glow upon our flying heroes from her mysterious throne in the starry night sky.

Day broke in tandem with a miraculous visage.

Crystalline waves rolled into one another and crashed against a creamy beach. Palm trees and flowers halted their approach toward the sea line when the soil turned to sand. From his position in the sky, Rom could see dolphins and mermaids playing in the water near the shore.

He was overcome with the majesty of such a vision. Blue was fast asleep atop the dragons back, doubled over his saddle. Rom dipped in the sky to wake the elf from his slumber. He knew that his plan had worked when he heard his friend gasp with delight at the sight in front of them.

Rom quickly landed right on the beach. A few of the mermaids covered their mouths in shock and darted underneath the water. He had forgotten for a moment that he was a dragon. He breathed deeply, taking in the smell and taste of the brackish air. Rom had always imagined the ocean would be beautiful, but in person, there was a profundity to the image.

Blue hopped off his friend's back and began looking around. He waved to a curious mermaid who smiled and returned the gesture. He approached the young mermaid and introduced himself and Rom. Her name was Cora, and she said that she had never met an elf or a dragon before. She was taken Rom and how majestic he looked standing in the sand before her beside his stately blue friend.

The three of them became deeply engaged in conversation, comparing, and contrasting their environments. Cora said that the sunsets on the beach were breathtaking, and they must stay to see one. The pair agreed and were not at all eager to make the journey back home. The young mermaid asked to see Rom breath fire. This was something that Rom had not mastered in the same way that his peers had, but he was willing to give it a try.

He turned toward the beach and tried to silence his thoughts. This was a technique that he had always used to maintain control over his emotions when he was anxious. He had discovered by accident one day that it also allowed him to focus his fire. Rom took a deep breath in through his nose and slowly let it out through his mouth. He found that if concentrated quite hard, something within his chest engaged with the breath, and it would turn into flames.

He was able to breathe out this fire toward the sand, and he watched as something miraculous happened. The areas where his breath had touched had turned clear and fluid. Rom had somehow fused the pieces of sand together under the heat of this exhalation.

Cora and Blue were just as shocked as the young dragon was. He had created something that they had never seen in their realm before, glass. They watched as the clear liquid hardened in a puddle. The dragon picked up a piece of this hardened glass because his skin was highly temperature resistant. He turned it over in his claws, in awe of the beauty of his creation.

Blue and Rom sat down immediately to brainstorm ways to use this new material. You could build things out of it, but it also seemed to shatter very easily. It was a stunning substance and could be used in any manner of art. The two shared ideas for the longest time, trying to decide how to approach this new object and its' potential usefulness. It was Blue on the beach that night, who came up with the idea of windows. The transparency it allowed was its most functional aspect.

The pair stayed to watch a coastal sunset with Cora, soaking up the natural beauty of their new favorite place. They packed up a sample of sand to bring to their communities so that they might demonstrate the usefulness of their discovery. They were hailed as inventors upon their return. The dragons and elves combined forces to set up a glass making operation right on the edge of the beach. Rom and Blue offered to travel there and oversee the production of the new material, as windows became one of the most in-demand items in all of Whimsy.

All of this took place a long, long time ago, and the people of Whimsy have been enjoying the benefits of the pairs trip for hundreds of years. They laid down the foundation for all sorts of new art and functional bowls, lightbulbs, windows, and even eventually mirrors. Mirrors being very important to a magical land filled with beautiful creatures. Every student in Whimsy learns the legend of Romulus and Blue.

As for our heroes, they traveled back and forth to the coast for their invention. They lived happily alongside their mermaid friend and their families back home. They served as an example of the good that can come from getting to know creatures that differ from yourself. They believed strongly in a free exchange of ideas among cultures. For the two best friends, this was just one of many adventures that they were fated to experience together as they split their time between the land they called home and the majestic sea.

Fighting Isn't Always the Answer

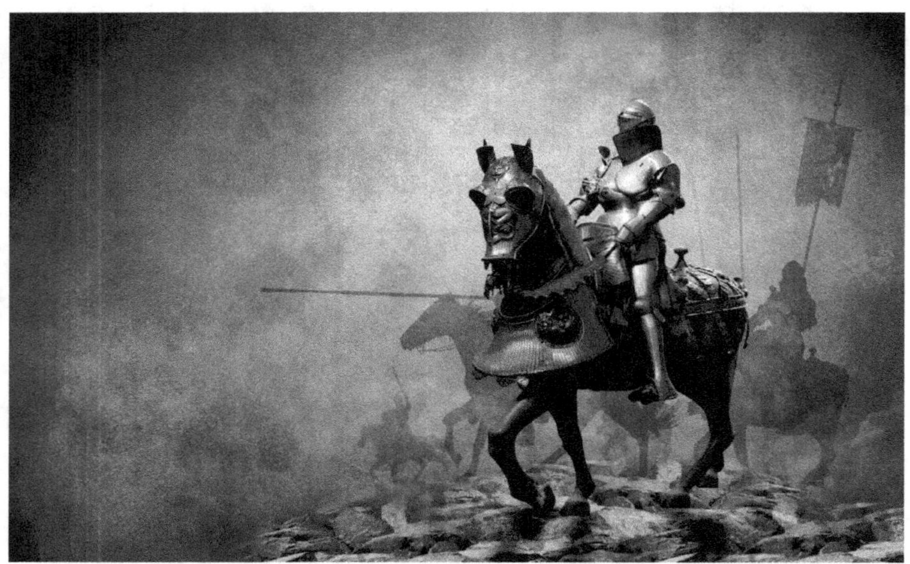

Arthur was a knight. He had his own convoy, or army, of knights and overall, it was a good group of knights. He had a squire named Alexander. Alexander was ready to become a knight and Arthur was planning the dubbing ceremony for after the next battle.

The convoy of knights was traveling through the countryside searching for a rogue band of knights. Arthur considered them rogue. They did not follow the Code of Chivalry and they were consistently breaking all the rules of conduct. Even though they pledged allegiance to the same liege lord, Knight Clifford needed to be taught a lesson and his convoy needed to be broken up. Arthur was taking the matter into his own hands. It troubled him little that he was possibly breaking the knight's code of chivalry because he was not breaking his own personal code. He felt that the world would be better without this group of marauding knights.

Arthur sent Alexander ahead to see how he does at scouting out the enemy camp. Arthur has seen signs all day that Clifford is slightly ahead of them but they are moving quickly and carelessly. Alexander should be seeing the same signs. Arthur will see just what skill Alexander has in finding the enemy. And then he will see what kind of strategy Alexander comes up with to invade the camp and conquer Clifford and the other knights. Alexander's brother, Calvin, had been squire to Clifford for some time but Clifford released him from service. Actually, Calvin was thrown out of the convoy. Though there were many reasons why Calvin would not make a good knight, Calvin was actually a perfect fit for Clifford and his convoy of knights.

Alexander returned in the middle of the night with news

of where Knight Clifford could be found. The large group was in a town nearby. They had basically invaded the town and were tormenting the residents by demanding food and drink.

"I can see the camp is spread out along a hillside," explained Alexander. "They have a good source of water, so they may be planning to stay for several days."

"Do you think we can battle them where they are right now?" asked Arthur.

"I think the hillside is would make it hard for a battle. Once the fighting starts, it will have to take place up the hill. The valley is narrow but it looks like the water is a little stream and would be easy to cross. It is lined with rocks, so it would be hard for horses to get across quickly."

Arthur asked about Clifford. "Where is Clifford? Does his squire seem to be organized and able?

Alexander thought about it for longer than Arthur expected. He finally answered, "Ay, his squire seems comfortable. I was watching the movement of the squire amongst the men. I think it is my brother, Calvin."

Arthur was a little surprised at this, but no totally. Calvin was with Clifford for a longer time than Alexander has been with Arthur. It would be hard to train someone new. Calvin may have been humiliated, but he was probably able to work his way back into the good humor of Clifford. He would probably just paid Clifford extra coin to be able to get back to being his squire. And Clifford probably wanted him back. They made a team.

"We will assume it is Calvin. What do you suggest we do? How should we take over the convoy?" asked Arthur. He wanted to know if Alexander was able to strategize and he would see how he is able to execute the strategy.

Alexander had been thinking about how to start a battle that would be a win for Arthur. He was thinking about it for the whole trip back to camp.

"I will go to the camp tomorrow with a list of ways they have not lived up to the Code of Chivalry. I am sure they will laugh in my face. I will then tell them that if they are not going to change, which I'm sure they won't, we will battle on a field just north of their camp on the following day. I will tell them it will be a fight to the finish."

Arthur understands that it must be this way, but he wants to be sure Alexander, and all the men, know that Clifford and his knights are not chivalrous and will fight until death. Arthur also knows The King likes Clifford because he always adds much gold to the King's coffers. The King does not care about chivalry and neither does Clifford. His men don't seem to care if they are chivalrous or not.

"Alexander, are you prepared for battle?" asked Arthur. This was not a question about whether the weapons were ready and the shields strong. This was about whether Alexander is ready to fight his brother.

"Sir, I am ready to serve you, my Liege," was Alexander's easy reply.

Arthur set about planning the battle. He knew the number of knights should not present a problem for him. There were several men in the ranks of Clifford's army that did not have a true loyalty to him. Arthur knew this because he had freed several men and knew Clifford's army was full of men who like to cause mayhem. They like to rob and steal and were not keen to fight. Arthur expected about 10 percent of the men to run off as soon as the trouble starts.

The men who stay to fight vary in terms of their abilities. Arthur noticed at the last tournament that the knights in Clifford's army have grown lazy and sloppy. They obviously did not practice with swords and lance. They were also, a lot of them, fat. Some have horses that seemed to strain under the weight of their master. Arthur planned to weed out the least skilled and push them to the side where they would be kept at bay by a few of his own men who were older and not able to fight for long periods of time. Arthur looked over to Alexander. Alexander was inspecting all weapons and shields that he and Arthur owned. This included things that had not been used in several years. Alexander felt that it was a waste to carry a weapon that was not in useful condition. Arthur had to agree with him.

Arthur was surprised to find Alexander sleeping that night. It appears that he is not worried about his plan to upset his brother and his brother's world. It was surprising, but Arthur was pleased. He picked the right boy to be his personal squire. The boy was now a man.

The next morning, Arthur had all the men gather around. Alexander was surprised when Arthur asked him to kneel and pledge his allegiance to the church and the king. Arthur then dubbed Alexander as a knight by touching his sword upon the shoulders of Alexander.

The men cheered and Alexander was pleased and surprised. He was expecting to be knighted after the battle. But there was work to be done and Alexander set out to do his part. He left to find Clifford and Calvin, knights of His Highness, the King. He entered the camp full of snorts and snores. Calvin was awake and checking his armor and looking for any issues with his chainmail. Alexander had done all of this as well, plus checking the armor and chainmail of Arthur. Alexander did not see Clifford, but he was here somewhere.

"Calvin. Where is your liege?" asked Alexander.

"Alex, I thought I felt you. It kept me up most of the night. Why are you here?"

"I am here to see your master. I have no quarrel with you. Not today, anyway."

"No quarrel with me? You are daft. I don't care if you have a quarrel with me. I have a quarrel with you. You left me humiliated on the field at the tourney. How could you do that to me, brother?"

"Oh, don't play the victim. You tried to cut my saddle so I would fall off my horse in the middle of the tournament. I have a true grievance. You fell off your horse by yourself. I was lucky to have found your sabotage before your games destroyed my life. Now, fetch me your liege," said Alexander in an angry voice Calvin had not heard before. His little brother was always showing a new side.

"Please, enough yelling!" yelled the liege, himself. I am trying to sleep here," came a drowsy voice from just behind Calvin.

"Sir Clifford, I bring a message from Sir Arthur."

"Because you have failed to uphold the Code of Chivalry and you do not live the life of a true knight, we challenge you to cease your nefarious behavior and uphold the values of which all knights are held to a high standard. Failure to do so will result in immediate physical removal of you and the knights of your allegiance. How say you, Sir?"

Clifford laughed. He laughed and laughed and laughed. He thought it was funny to have a boy tell him what to do and how to behave.

When Clifford was done laughing, he spat at Alexander. He missed his mark, but Alexander understood the sentiment.

"Tomorrow at sunrise, Sir. The battle shall begin tomorrow at sunrise."

Alexander rode back to his own camp. He took a direct route and did little to conceal his travel. He tried to make it seem that he did not know Calvin would follow him, but he knew he would. That is why he did not even bother to say where the battle would take place. He discussed it with Arthur before he left and Arthur agreed. Clifford and Calvin would not fight fairly. They would rather ambush the camp than follow code to fight fairly. This is precisely why they need to be stopped.

Arthur had been following out of sight to make a note of how many men were set to fight against him and his knights. So far, it was only Calvin. Calvin was moving stealthily. He did not want to be seen. When Calvin was close to Arthur's camp, he turned around and returned to Clifford. Arthur followed him to try to get an understanding of their plot.

"Calvin, how many men are there?" asked Clifford.

"I counted 20. It is a small group. It will not be a problem to overtake them if we go now before the rest of the knights come back from town."

Arthur listened to the two talking and was expecting them to put a little more thought into the plot against him. They were just going to wake up a few men and take them to fight a battle against the "unsuspecting" knights.

Arthur was sure there would be more to the plot and so he followed them as they rode with a total of twelve men in full armor on their warhorses. Alexander was in charge of getting the men ready at the camp. It was true that there were only a few men at the camp when Calvin saw them, but the others were simply lounging on the other side of the hill. They should all be ready for battle now, ready to disband the evil in the most permanent way.

Calvin and Clifford did not notice the quiet that was settling around them. The birds were not chirping because they flew away when the men settled in the branches of the trees. One by one, the men leaped out of the trees and landed on the backs of Clifford's men as they passed beneath. The men in the trees were not in armor. They were a lot more mobile than the men dressed for battle. The knights knocked the armored soldiers off their warhorses and someone on the ground knocked the man unconscious with a large mallet. Because they were in armor, Clifford and Calvin did not hear all of the commotion going on around them. They were riding fast and it was until they were the only two left they realized something was very wrong.

By this time, Arthur and Alexander were riding side by side toward Clifford and Calvin. I would be a duel between the four of them, knight against knight, brother against brother. Shields were lowered and lances were readied and they charge at each other. There were maces swinging and the lances were used to know the riders from astride the horses. The noise was deafening. Alexander knocked Calvin off balance with his lance then turned back and hit Calvin with the mace in his shoulder. Calvin tried to raise his shield but he was too late. He was heading to the ground. Clifford was not having better luck. His mace had fallen to the ground after the lance brushed him with more force than he was prepared to take. Though he was still on his horse, he was shaken. It was not to be believed. He thought of all the tricks he has used in the past. He had many, but he needed Calvin next to him to pull them off. Calvin was not there. He is on the ground and he isn't moving. There isn't any blood, but the side of his helmet is bashed in quite badly. Tired of wasting time and not sure where his men were, Clifford decided to flee back to his camp.

Clifford's camp was not controlled by the knights of Arthur. They took over the camp. The rowdy knights were corralled into a quickly made cage. It was Alexander's idea on a previous campaign to have everything they need to set up a large cage for prisoners. It works very well and they had the laziest of the knights locked inside. Some of the knights fled. They were followed and they appear to have no intention of fighting. They are simply running away. Around the time the sun was setting, Clifford came racing back to the camp. He was surprised to see his knights caged like the animals at The Colosseum. "What a disappointment," he thought. "You can't count on anyone, not even yourself." Calvin was still not awake. He was kicked in the head by his horse after he fell. Both Calvin and Clifford were stripped of their armor and weapons. Their clothes were inspected and their boots removed. There were many weapons hidden in their clothes and boots. They were truly ready to fight to the death. Instead of death, they were placed inside the cage with the other knights where they stayed until a tournament was organized and the men were paraded through the tournament grounds while a list of offenses against the Code of Chivalry was read. Many of the townspeople they had harmed were there to see their shame. They would never be accepted as knights again.

Alexander was a good and strong knight. He formed a convoy of young soldiers and they vowed to abide by the Code of Chivalry and to protect the Church and the King. They killed as few soldiers as possible, but they did as they must in the name of their liege lord. The problem they saw was that battles were won; the loser regrouped and came back to fight again. It was a cycle that just kept happening again and again. Alexander and his soldiers made sure to be alert and have weapons ready so they would always be ready for an attack. It was the choice they made, to love God and to fight. So that is what they did. They served their King well, always bringing coin from the sale of armor and weapons. They did what they could to destroy the weapons of the men defeated on the battlefield. They hoped it would deter the survivors from setting out to fight again. The usually found more money to buy more weapons and challenged the King's knights again. The circle of fighting battles is never-ending.

A Pyramid Discovery

A long time ago, there lived a king. His name was King Toba. King Toba was generally a good king. He reigned justly, and therefore it was hard for his people to be hard complaining. King Toba valued hard work and honesty, and he urged his people to adopt these virtues. Every morning during the peaceful time, he will lead his people in cultivating various cross for food. He firmly believed that his people would be vulnerable without food. So as a result, the food stores were always full of the trim with the grain. People were happy.

King Toba also had a beautiful daughter, princess Lia. The princess was so gorgeous that whenever she passed, the king's square everyman would stop to wonder at her exceptional beauty. She was also very respectful and friendly. However, the princess was the apple of her father's eyes and was therefore well guarded. No man was ever allowed anywhere near her without direct permission from the father.

So, it happened that the was one young man called Tibe. Tibe was the blacksmith. He was so skilled at his work that sometimes he would win the praise of the king. Tibe's interest, it would appear, was not only in working on sturdy iron. He was also interested in the princess. He was so much in love with her. He dreamt about her every day. And when he told his mother, the mother dismissed him

"mother, one day I will marry the princess, "he will begin. The mother will smile inwardly and then say, "my son, please don't aim at the sun when the gods intended you to reside on the moon. Look for a nice girl, your status, and marry her. The princess is not for you."

"But I love her so much mother, what shall I do?" Tibe would ask.

"There are other beautiful girls around who admire you Tibe. Look at Han's daughter, beautiful, hardworking, and respectful. And I know for a fact that the girl loves you. Look at the way she looks at you. Marry her and forget all about the princess."

Although he was popular with the girls, he couldn't find any girl who resembled his dream girl, the princes. He had to find a way. He had to. He then resumed his work, but his mind was racing with many thoughts. He was wondering how to attract the princess' attention. He decided the next time she passed through the square; he will present her with flowers. He might find a chance to talk to her. But he knew it would be difficult bearing in mind the mean guards who always accompanied her wherever they went.

He knew the princess would be touring the square on the following day. So, with his savings, he went to the flower shop at the corner. He wanted to buy the best flowers available.

"I need flowers, the best available. Flowers that can talk to a girl, "he asked the shop attendant.

"Any special occasion?"

"yes, there is this girl, whom I love greatly need to

impress her tomorrow morning," he replied wryly.

"Well, there are flowers. Then there are special flowers. But since you are not using them today, why don't you come in the morning. Let me prepare the special ones for you."

Tibe then paid for the flowers. He will pick them the following day then wait for the princess to arrive. He was starting to feel confident. He hoped the girl would like him. He prayed.

The following morning, he woke up very early, and he was at the flower shop even before it opened. The shop attendant was surprised to find him standing there.

"morning prince charming, I can see you are already up," the attendant greeted him cheerfully.

"Yes, as you know, our forefathers warn us that man should wake up ahead of the sun. that is why I am here this early," Tibe replied.

"True, my friend. A man who loves sleep always invites Poverty through the windows. Anyway, your flowers are ready, let me show you," the attendant said.

Once inside, Tibe was presented with the most beautiful flowers his eyes had ever seen. Not that he was an expert in the knowledge of flowers, but he knew a lovely flower when he saw one.

"my friend. I had to get this beautiful flower for you after hearing about your mission later today. This flower carries luck. Go and present it to the girl of your dream. You wot come back disappointed, "the attendant explained

Tube thanked him profusely and headed out to the square, the flowers on his hand. He didn't know the time the princess will come. So, he sat down and waited. He waited and waited but still the princess as nowhere. He waited some more, but the princess didn't come out of the palace. He was about to give up when he glimpsed the familiar chariots of the palace's first family coming from a distance. He stood up and squinted his eyes towards it. He hoped it was the princess' chariot.

His heart started pounding hard as the chariot drew near and nearer. It was indeed the princess being driven around the kingdom. He recognized the princess's flag, which was always mounted on the leading chariot. There was a problem though. It was simply impossible to walk up to the princess without passing through the guards. He quickly thought up an idea, but none was forthcoming. So, he did the craziest thin no sane man would do.

He jumped in the middle of the way, blocking the chariots' way and shouted the princess' name

"princess Lia! "he shouted so loudly that everyone stopped doing what they were doing and turned to look at the Youngman in the middle of the road. His shout was also heard by the princess, who looked through the window only to find an energetic man with flowers on his hand.

 She didn't know what to make of it correctly. And his actions brought the wrath of the overzealous guards who descendent on him with fists and blows. But Tibe was so determined. He fought his way to the princess' carriage and threw the flowers to her. The flowers landed on her seat. She picked the flowers and smelled. It had a pleasant smell. She next stepped out and ordered the guards to leave Tibe alone.

"Am so sorry my princess to come to you this way," Tibe said

"What is your name?" asked the princess.

"I am Tibe. The blacksmith. Please accept my flowers."

"Thank you for the flowers. And for your troubles, I invite you to the princess' party next week at the king's palace. I will keep the flowers," the princess replied. And the chariot moved on.

Tibe was injured, but he seemed not to feel any pain. He was so happy with himself for accomplishing the mission. He was exalted at the invitation of the princess. He hoped she liked the flower. He walked very fast to his home. He had to let his skeptical mother know about the good news. He found his mother kneading bread. She immediately stood up in alarm.

"What happened to you, did you have an accident," she asked.

"no mother, there was no accident. I met the princess..." he started explaining, but his mother cut him off.

"I knew it. That princess will kill you," she said and then rushed inside to pick the healing oil which she administered gently on Tibe's wounds.

"mother, I met her today. She is adorable. And she invited me to her party," Tibe explained.

"She did what?' Her mother asked. She was surprised at the turn of events. But still, she didn't want Tibe associating with the mighty princess. She reasoned that such actions would only lead to her being hurt. But her son was getting obsessed with the princess with each passing day. She didn't know how best to stop him.

Meanwhile, in the palace, the princess placed the flowers on the table next to her dressing mirror. She just loved the smell of the flowers. It was so unique. She had never seen such adorable flowers, and she kept wondering where it came from. That night, when she slept, she dreamt the flowers had grown into a big umbrella, and she was flying around the kingdom while holding the knob. The experience was magical, and when she woke up from the dream, she walked to the dressing table and picked the flowers and smelt again. She then returned to bed, and soon she was deep asleep.

When she woke up the following morning, she was surprised to find the flowers fresh again as if it had just been picked straight from the field. Usually, her flowers would wilt within a day. But these flowers remained fresh for days, and so was its smell. Questions rang in her mind, but the only person who could answer was the man who presented her with the flowers. She told herself she would have to inquire more about the flower from the palace's servants.

She summoned some of the experienced servants to try and explain all they knew about the flower, which never wilted. But no one seems to know anything about that particular flower. No one had ever seen the flower before. She decided to wait for the princess party, which was due in a week. She hoped the young man who presented her with the flowers would turn up. From then on, the princess carried the flowers wherever she went. It was observed that she was getting obsessed with the flowers. She ate better, laughed better, and was happier when she had the flowers on her hand.

Back to Tibe. The boy was simply over the moon. His mind was focused on meeting the princess again. He wondered what to wear to the party. He also wondered how he would best behave in the palace. He had heard that the king never condoned some behaviors from those around him. His mother, however, was concerned with the boy. He seemed to find interest in no one or anything else. He was not eating well anymore. He even failed to report at work once or twice that week. This was something that had never happened before.

Finally, the day of the party arrived. Tibe woke up very early. He took a long slow bath then dressed in the impeccable brand-new clothes he had bought a few days ago. The clothes had cost him an arm and a leg. He headed for the palace immediately after breakfast. On arriving at the gate, he was informed that the party was for that evening and he had come a little earlier. He was then told to wait outside until the event started. He sat outside the palace gates and waited for hours. And finally, his long wait bore fruits. The gates were opened at exactly four in the evening.

Tibe, with everyone else who had been invited, stepped into the palace in awe. The building was beautiful and clean. It was a vast place with countless servants who seemed to carry out their duties in a seamless pattern. They were directed to the ball area room, the location of the party. They were served with drinks and various food. They enjoyed some music pelted out by a live performance band. Food and beverages were in plenty.

As the party progressed, more and more guests arrived, including the prince of the neighborhood kingdom. Prince Charles was rumored to have an interest in the princess. The prince had proposed to the princess once or twice, but his offer was turned down. The princess needed time, but the prince was getting impatient. He intended to see the king's help to convince her daughter to marry him.

Soon the first family's arrival was announced, and everybody offered their welcoming clap. Tibe, for the first time that day, saw the princess. She was so beautiful and adorable. The princess was wearing a beautiful white gown, and on her hand, to Tibe's delight, she was holding the unique flowers he had given her several days earlier. Tibe wondered how the princess had managed to keep the flowers fresh and beautiful for days.

The king then gave out his speech to the crowd. He welcomed them to his daughter's event and reminded everyone about the need to maintain peace and harmony in the kingdom. He repeated his clarion call of the need for hard work. After that, he welcomed everyone to the dance floor. This was the moment Tibe had been waiting for. Feeling confident, perhaps from the several glasses of wine he'd had droned, he told himself he must find a way to dance with the princess. He knew it was not easy, but there was always away.

The princess was also secretly scanning the cord for Tibe, the flower man, but she seems to be having trouble locating him. After several attempts, she finally discovered him. He was dancing awkwardly alone in the middle of the dance floor. She moved to where he was.

"Hello, care for a dance?" she asked, startling him.

"Princess, ooh sure," then they headed for the floor. As they were dancing, the princess asked him several questions, but of most interests to her was the flower. She wanted to know where Tibe had fetched it from.

"A friend gave me. It is a special flower," Tibe replied.

"Yes, I love it so much it is now my companion," replied the princess. Tibe was so pleased to hear the princess say that. They danced some more and soon the party was over. They had to part.

That night, the princess couldn't trace her favorite flower. It had just disappeared mysteriously during the party. Someone must have kept it for her. The following morning, she summoned all her servants, but nobody seemed to have seen the flower. A frenzied search was carried out in all the chambers of the palace, but still, no flower was found. Several days of searching bore no fruit.

Then the princess became depressed over it. She wanted her flower. She refused to eat or talk to anyone. The king and the queen became concerned for their daughter. So, the king ordered an investigation to be done on the source of the flower. And soon, the flower was traced to Tibe, who was summoned to the king's palace. He, however, explained he bought the flower from the flower shop. The king ordered the attendant to be summoned, but when the guards reached the shop, it was closed, and there was no sign of the attendant. He, too, like the flower was missing.

Meanwhile, the princess's condition was getting worse by the day. After several days of not eating, she collapsed into a coma.

The king, in his desperation, made a declaration. Whoever will find the unique flower will marry her daughter. Tibe swore to use all his power to find the flower. He thought of the best way to locate it. And so, he spent several days thinking and searching for the flower with no success.

One day as he was buried in sleep, he had a strange dream. He dreamed he was inside the Pharaoh's pyramid situated several miles away. And while inside, he came across thousands of the unique flowers like the one he had presented the princess. The following morning, he woke up early and headed for the pyramid. After walking for hours, he finally arrived. He entered inside and started the search. After searching every room, he couldn't locate the flower. Tired, he decided to sit down and rest next to a big statue of a lion. He was dozing off when the statue started to talk to him,

"Tibe, I will help you find the flower if you help me," the lion statue said in a clear voice, startling Tibe. His first instinct was to flee, but he then thought of the princess and her suffering.

"How can I help you?" he finally gathered enough courage to ask.

"Simple, touch at my brow, and I will come back to life again. That is the only way I will defeat the spell," the statue said. It explained that a terrible witch had cast a spell on him and ever since it was turned into a statue.

The moment Tibe touched the brow of the lion, the statue changed first into a lion, then into a man. The man then led Tibe into a hidden room where several flowers like the one the princess was looking or were growing. He Picked several of them, thanked the man, and quickly rushed to the palace.

The king received the flower cheerfully and took it to the princess' room. He ordered the flower to be given to the princess to smell. She regained her consciousness immediately; she sniffed the flower. She was starving, and after eating to her full, she asked for Tibe.

Several days later, the princess fully recovered, and soon the king allowed Tibe to marry her. They lived happily after that. And that is how Tibe discovered the flowers which never wilted inside the pyramid.

Conclusion

In summary, this book acknowledges that the reader is looking for a solution and is already disturbed by the difficulties of not getting sleep or not realizing quality sleep. The author makes an effort to present guidelines, proven guidelines, of how to attain guided meditation to overcome anxiety and insomnia that adversely affect the sleep patterns and the duration of sleep. The book systematically addresses guided meditation to induce children to sleep. The layout and the flow of the book are meant to allow the user to benefit from whichever chapter that the reader starts with. However, the author recommends the audience reading through from the first chapter to the last chapter.

Lack of sleep and lack of quality sleep affects the physical, physiological and mental health status of children. In this manner, lack of sleep and lack of quality sleep can lead to anger, irritability, and lack of concentration when executing routine duties which can be dangerous. The meditation scripts given in this book are itemized and simple enough to suit children engaging in guided hypnosis or guided meditation for the first time including seasoned kids with respect to meditation.

Meditation are excellent tools for helping your children feel more confident, creative, and relaxed. At its necessary foundation, just sitting still and quiet for a length of time is a powerful tool. This space that you create for them ignites their imagination and focus on just breathing. It also gives them a time and place to feel their emotions. It is also a message to them that feeling, expressing, and talking about their views is a good thing. Meditation also gives children the chance to be their true selves, even when all the other time in the day they may feel like they need to act or say or be a different way. In the space of meditation, your child can be whoever they are or want to be. That is a powerful moment to give!

The meditations you and your children are about to go through are a mixture of techniques to reach children in different ways. Focus on sounds, breathing, or a specific thought aids your children to start developing essential skills to help their coping and their focus skills as they continue growing. Besides, every meditation script presents a chance for your children to demonstrate their creativity through imaginations and visualizations. They provide compelling images to picture in their minds as the intended message and support sink deep in their brains.